Et~~hical~~

D A T~~E DUE~~

D0732309

This book is due on the last date sta~~mped~~
wi~~th~~

# Ethical Responsibility in Pharmacy Practice

## Robert A. Buerki, Ph.D.

Professor
Division of Pharmacy Practice and Administration

The Ohio State University

## Louis D. Vottero, M.S.

Professor of Pharmacy Emeritus

Ohio Northern University

American Institute of the History of Pharmacy
Madison, Wisconsin
2002

**Acknowledgments:** Pages 208-10: "Principles of Medical Ethics" and "Fundamental Elements of the Patient-Physician Relationship," reprinted with permission from the Code of Medical Ethics, American Medical Association, © 1994 and © 2000. AMA logo reprinted with the permission of the American Medical Association. © 2002 American Medical Association. Usage of the AMA logo does not imply an endorsement of the non-AMA material found in this book.

Page 211: "Code of Ethics for Nurses with Interpretive Statements," reprinted with permission from the American Nurses Association, © 2001 American Nurses Publishing, American Nurses Foundation/American Nurses Association, Washington, D.C.

Pages 212-15: "A Patient's Bill of Rights," reprinted with permission of the American Hospital Association, © 1992.

Pages 216-17: "Pharmacy Patient's Bill of Rights," reprinted with permission of the National Association of Boards of Pharmacy.

**On the cover:** The "triad of medical care" has been the basis for the ethical relationship between the pharmacist, the physician, and the patient for centuries. In the background, an early depiction of the triad from Book 7 of the encyclopedia *On the Properties of Things* by Bartholomew the Englishman, published in Westminster about 1495. In the foreground, a photograph of a contemporary triad (courtesy of the Department of Veterans Affairs).

**Cover design:** Robert A. Buerki and Cynthia A. Gray

# CONTENTS

# TABLE OF CASES

# INTRODUCTION TO THE SECOND EDITION

In the decade since this little textbook was conceived, the American practice of pharmacy has undergone a profound sea change. In the early 1990s, pharmacy educators were still debating whether the entry-level Pharm.D. should be a universal requirement; Congress briefly considered, then quickly dropped, a plan which would have provided the United States with national health insurance, including a prescription benefit; "pharmaceutically assisted death" became a reality in Oregon; OBRA '90 brought legislative grit to the ethical mandate for patient counseling by pharmacists; and the American Pharmaceutical Association established a broad-based committee to develop a code of ethics for all pharmacists. Riding the crest of these waves was the new practice philosophy of pharmaceutical care, so full of professional promise, yet untested in everyday pharmacy practice.

All these changes brought a new interest and urgency to the teaching of professional ethics in our schools and colleges of pharmacy. The AACP's Commission to Implement Change in Pharmaceutical Education included "facility with values and ethical principles" in its statement of general educational outcomes, which were given added importance when adopted as accreditation criteria by the American Council on Pharmaceutical Education; the handful of elective courses that had survived the curricular crunch of the 1990s were dusted off and given new life; our friend and colleague, Amy Haddad, organized a brilliant series of workshops for teachers of pharmacy ethics, including one on the ethics of pharmaceutical care; the American Association of Colleges of Pharmacy supported the creation of an Ethics Special Interest Group (SIG); new textbooks on pharmacy ethics (including this one) appeared on the market; the Code of Ethics for Pharmacists was ratified by members of the American Pharmaceutical Association in 1994 and offered to the profession.

By the end of the decade, the Doctor of Pharmacy degree was the standard entry-level preparation for pharmacy practice; as the baby-boom generation settled into retirement and anecdotage, the demand for prescriptions approached and then exceeded 3 billion orders annually; schools and colleges of pharmacy could not

xi

graduate enough pharmacists to meet the demand, and the institutions themselves reproduced at a rate no one would have predicted ten years earlier; pharmacy technicians graduated from certified programs and were licensed in some states, adding a new fillip to the pharmacy manpower problem; mail-order prescription programs, once dismissed as an annoyance, now set industry standards for speed and reliability in a multibillion-dollar prescription market; direct-to-consumer prescription drug advertising soared and Internet "pharmacies" thrived, giving consumers unprecedented freedom in the choice of their therapy; advanced computer software and robotics promised to free the pharmacist's time to counsel patients, but the OBRA-mandated "offer to counsel" was still too often observed in its breach; the notion of pharmaceutical care has been embraced by the profession, but the practice philosophy still struggles in its implementation, as deep-discount pharmacy chains continue to believe that all the American public wants from its pharmacists is good, cheap prescription drugs delivered up as quickly as possible; and the Code of Ethics for Pharmacists has yet to be universally adopted by the pharmacy profession, as it struggles once again to redefine its societal purpose.

This new edition of *Ethical Responsibility in Pharmacy Practice* includes new sections on controversial topics such as terminal sedation, euthanasia, and assisted suicide; ethical issues associated with controlling prices on prescription medication; and the ethical challenges presented by alternative medications. A commentary has been added to each case study, which pharmacy students should find useful as they develop their own set of professional practice values and methods of resolving the ethical conflicts they will face in their professional practice; an extensive glossary of terms also has been added as a courtesy to the reader. Our educational goal, however, stated in 1994, remains the same: "By introducing students to ethical concepts, giving them directed practice in applying ethical principles, and allowing them to develop skills in problem-solving and critical thinking, the instructor of professional ethics can heighten student sensitivity, increase professional awareness, and, indirectly, improve health care at the critical pharmacist-patient interface."

# INTRODUCTION TO THE FIRST EDITION

America appears to have been foundering in an ethical crisis for the past several years. As individuals in the highest ranks of government, the clergy, business, and sports became caught in a quagmire of lies, sharp dealing, impropriety, and scandal, Americans began to reexamine the underlying moral tenets in our society and found them wanting. Politicians charged that educators condoned and even fostered a plurality of values in our school systems; educators pointed to the decline in church attendance as the root of the problem; and clergy blamed the government for removing moral teachings from public education on overly zealous Constitutional grounds. At the same time, the American health-care system underwent its most tortuous redefinition in recent history as third parties started to examine quality of care, professional competence, allocation of resources, and to insist upon health maintenance, all within the pervading aura of cost-containment. Finally, an increasingly sophisticated public demanded that its health care be not only more affordable, but virtually flawless in its outcomes. The alternative, it declared, was litigation, and malpractice insurance rates soared.

Throughout this turmoil, American pharmacy emerged remarkably unscathed. Its practitioners basked in the warm glow of public trust and confidence and continued to expand patient services. Pharmacy educators began to stress interpersonal communication skills in their already crowded curricula in an attempt to enhance patient care through improved compliance with prescribed medication. Yet as patient communication increased, the nagging ethical issues of preserving patient confidentiality and autonomy while maintaining openness and truthfulness tested the resourcefulness of pharmacy practitioners and students alike. To be sure, pharmacy ethics has traditionally held a small place in the scheme of pharmaceutical education, if only relegated to a dean intoning the APhA Code of Ethics to his senior pharmacy students on the eve of their graduation. Yet by the mid-1970s, court decisions had seriously eroded the role of codes of ethics in maintaining standards of professional practice beyond that required by law and had brought into question the role that peer review should play in ensuring a collective self-discipline. Faced with uncertain alternatives and what they perceived to be a crumbling of the nation's moral foundations, pharmacy educators began looked at formal instruction in professional ethics with new interest and commitment. At the same time, leaders in pharmacy practice called for a review of the profession's code of ethics, requesting the APhA to spearhead the development of a new "Code of Ethics for Pharmacists." *Ethical Responsibility in Pharmacy Practice* is the result of this interest and commitment; it would not have been published five years ago.

Instruction in professional ethics in a school or college of pharmacy poses several unusual challenges: To the student inured to scientific facts, reproducible laboratory values, and precise measurements, the study of ethics seems maddeningly arbitrary, a gray morass of competing principles that intrude upon a black-and-white world of unquestioned facts. Moreover, the student must not only master ethical principles, but learn to choose among alternatives and resolve ethical dilemmas at the higher level of abstraction represented by such problem-solving skills. To the instructor who cannot typically claim expertise in moral philosophy at the graduate level and may not be intimately familiar with the ethical dilemmas that plague today's pharmacy practitioners, the teaching of ethics may prove an uncomfortable, even threatening assignment, particularly in the give-and-take arena of small-group discussion. Moreover, the instructor may feel uneasy in taking a personal stand on ethical issues discussed in the classroom setting. Finally, the administrator who feels obliged to include required instruction in ethics in an already overcrowded undergraduate pharmacy curriculum is often caught between the specter of tokenism and the equally unattractive alternative of eliminating or compromising other course work.

The authors have had the luxury of testing out their ideas by teaching professional ethics to small groups of interested pharmacy students in elective proseminars over the past two decades. Upper-division pharmacy students who have had at least a modicum of practical experience in either the hospital or the community setting seem to profit most from weekly two-hour proseminars. While lectures are useful in conveying basic ethical principles, small-group discussions of no more than twenty-five students are necessary to develop the skills of critical thinking and problem-solving upon which intelligent ethical decision-making is based. Moreover, the students learn to become tolerant to a wide range of opinion from their contemporaries, which enhances the learning situation. Although this book has been primarily designed as a text for free-standing courses in pharmacy ethics, teachers of jurisprudence, dispensing, or clinical practice may wish to use it as a companion text to introduce basic concepts of applied ethical decision-making. Moreover, preceptors in externship and clerkship settings can use the text to complement their individual mentoring of advanced pharmacy students prior to graduation.

The authors strongly believe that trends in professional values and ethical standards can be understood best within the historical context of American pharmacy practice. For example, while older versions of professional codes of ethics mirror changes in professional practices over time, reflecting changes in educational standards, legal obligations, and professional functions, the newly adopted Code of Ethics for Pharmacists reflects a fundamental shift to an ethos based upon morals and virtues. Accordingly, this text has been designed to reflect the developmental changes in the practice of pharmacy over the past century and to account for the transformation in professional values and ethics engendered by these changes. The ethical issues associated with each topical area considered—pharmacist-patient relationships, professional communications, and drug distribution—have also been developed within their own unique historical contexts.

While the teaching of professional ethics is undoubtedly labor-intensive, it can also be deeply satisfying: By introducing students to ethical concepts, giving them directed practice in applying ethical principles, and allowing them to develop skills in problem-solving and critical thinking, the instructor of professional ethics can heighten student sensitivity, increase professional awareness, and, indirectly, improve health care at the critical pharmacist-patient interface. *Ethical Responsibility in Pharmacy Practice* is our modest contribution to these goals.

# CHAPTER 1

# PROFESSIONAL VALUES IN PHARMACY PRACTICE

The traditional function of pharmacy practice—compounding and dispensing medications directly to the public in a safe and reliable manner—predates the emergence of the pharmacy profession itself. In every age and in every culture, individuals have taken the rather awesome responsibility for learning about and preparing medicines for others and, in a sense, managing their health care. The practice of pharmacy and, indeed, all healing professions is an intensely personal, peculiarly human activity that has been traditionally guided by such basic human values as compassion, dignity, justice, and truth. In recent times, the importance of these values has been underscored by surgical virtuosity, the prospect of pharmacogenomic drugs, and other dazzling technical innovations that have revolutionized modern medical and pharmaceutical practice.

Although human values are more commonly associated with such humanistic disciplines as philosophy and religion, health professionals are beginning to realize that the success of their medical interventions with their patients depends as much upon interpersonal, value-based relationships as it does upon technical competence. When the full range of personal and societal values associated with pharmacy practice is taken into consideration, even the seemingly benign activity of recommending a nonprescription medication takes on added meaning. Rather than making a quick clinical judgment and recommending a product, pharmacists sensitive to their patients' individual needs may defer a "sale," recommend medical intervention, suggest a change in life style, or just offer comfort and reassurance. To what extent, for example, does the perceived socioeconomic status of the patient determine the extent and nature of the professional services pharmacists provide? To what extent do the pressures for cost-containment influence the pharmacist's drug-product selection process? How does the acceptance of the practice philosophy of pharmaceutical care affect the value system of American pharmacists? Indeed, human values seem to be so completely integrated with modern health-care practices, that one might argue that the so-called "ideal" of a highly technical, purely clinical, and "value-free" practice of medicine or pharmacy is neither possible nor even desirable. Thus, any vaunted claim of "value neutrality" in contemporary health-care practices may be no more than a tolerance for a plurality of values or, worse, an excuse to avoid dealing with ethical dilemmas altogether. We must, however, remember the uniqueness of individual personal value systems: our righteous indignation over colleagues who appear to be avoiding moral responsibility very well may be a reaction to the unsettling possibility that they do not hold our values.

## Traditional professional values in pharmacy practice

By the end of the nineteenth century, the practice of pharmacy in the United States emerged as a socially necessary function, distinct from medicine, and sanctioned by society. These sanctions took the form of licensure laws and examination procedures that established a benchmark for professional pharmacy practice. Turn-of-the-century pharmacists not only fulfilled their professional function of compounding and dispensing physicians' prescriptions, but also served as self-appointed guardians and advisors, dedicated to protecting their customers from dangerous poisons or fraudulent patent medicines. In some hospitals and other institutions, a handful of pharmacists manufactured irrigating solutions and prepared other drug products in bulk as their primary activity. In neighborhood drugstores, most pharmacists subsidized their professional function by selling other drug-related items and a wide range of so-called "lines"—cosmetics, tobaccos, sodas, sundries, and other unrelated commodities in an essentially mercantile setting. These pharmacists displayed a genuine concern for their patrons, dispensing simple drugs, patent medicines, and homely health-care advice to a trusting, unsophisticated clientele, earning their respect and the sobriquet "Doc." The basic value of pharmacy practice was built upon personal service, which affirmed pharmacists' belief in themselves as health-care professionals.

In burgeoning colleges of pharmacy, avuncular pharmacist-professors emphasized the identification, assaying, and testing of drug products, and the careful weighing, compounding, and dispensing of prescriptions. By the mid-1930s, universally required baccalaureate programs in pharmacy sought to infuse a well-rounded general education into the traditional professional curriculum, a strategy calculated to result in both professional and public respect. "Your pharmacist is the scientist on the corner," public relations campaigns of the period proudly proclaimed. Licensure boards began to supervise components of practice through internship programs, a remnant of the traditional apprenticeship system of training. In the corner drugstore, good pharmaceutical service was defined in terms of elegantly prepared drug products with neatly-typed labels; hospital pharmacists stocked "drug rooms" from which doctors and nurses could obtain the drugs their patients needed. At about the same time, pharmaceutical manufacturers began to market more effective and sophisticated finished dosage forms that did not require further compounding by individual practitioners. Many pharmacists, however, resisted this technological intrusion and continued to cling to their limited vision of pharmaceutical service, bounded by the traditional compounding and distributive functions. Others even sought to increase this function by promoting so-called U.S.P. and N.F. "propaganda" campaigns through their state pharmaceutical associations. These campaigns encouraged physicians to write prescriptions for formulas in the official compendia that pharmacists could extemporaneously compound instead of merely dispensing the commercially available versions of the same products.[1] Certain groups of pharmacists continue to resist external challenges to their comfortable practice environments. As we will see, mail-order pharmacy operations, prescription insurance programs, and mandated patient counseling spark debates among today's pharmacists as stirring as the struggle to maintain the compounding function of sixty years ago.

By the early 1940s, drug therapy continued to evolve from palliative, symptomatic treatments to specific, effective chemotherapeutic agents. The focus of the pharmacist's professional function in all settings began to shift from the extemporaneous compounding of simple drug products to the increasingly efficient, cost-effective dispensing of dosage forms prepared by large, specialized pharmaceutical manufacturers. In teaching hospitals and other institutions, rededicated to therapeutic effectiveness and better patient services, a growing number of committed pharmacists defined the first practice specialty in pharmacy, one which began to focus upon serving individual patient needs through a system of optimum drug distribution.[2]

In the community setting, the concepts of self-service and mass merchandising redefined first chain and then independent

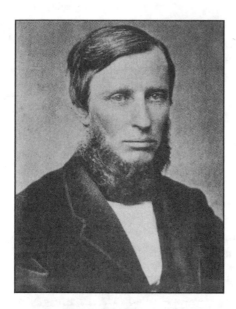

Edward Parrish (1822-72), author of the 1857 essay "Ethical Analysis," possibly the first serious consideration of American pharmacists' moral responsibilities. (*Kremers Reference Files, F. B. Power Pharmaceutical Library, University of Wisconsin-Madison.*)

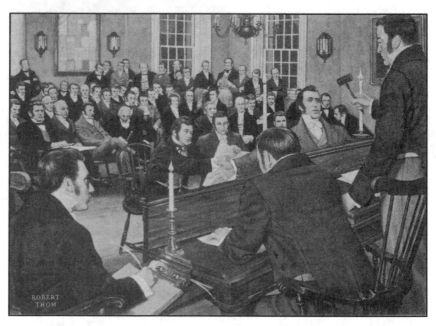

In 1848 the Philadelphia College of Pharmacy promulgated the first American code of ethics for pharmacists. The painting "American Pharmacy Builds Its Foundations" by Robert Thom shows the artist's conception of the founding of the College in 1821. (*Illustration courtesy of Parke-Davis, division of Warner Lambert.*)

pharmacy practice, just as they had redefined the grocery and department stores of the 1930s. The steady growth of aggressive drugstore chains, which often considered their prescription departments as just another "line," frustrated many independent pharmacy practitioners. Some simply attempted to compete head-on with the chains in disastrous price-cutting wars; other more professionally minded pharmacists tried to promote their prescription departments while still providing the wide range of merchandise and services that had come to characterize the American drugstore. Despite the sweeping societal changes swirling about them, pharmacists continued to cling to their traditional service value. In their zeal to "serve the public," pharmacists added new "lines," provided free delivery for minor purchases, opened family charge accounts, sold postage stamps, and maintained mind-numbing sixteen-hour work days, seven days a week, providing the high level of service they felt the public expected from their corner drugstore.[3]

In this product-centered practice, professional values were dominated by service and accuracy. Pharmacists provided quick, attentive service and accurately prepared drug products for their patients, most of whom they usually referred to as "patrons" or "customers." Pharmacists prided themselves on the warm, interpersonal relationships they established with their patients, but refrained from taking any active responsibility for their health care, merely recommending either physician intervention or only the most benign over-the-counter remedies. To do otherwise, that is, to engage in so-called "counter-prescribing," would have encroached upon the physician's prerogative to diagnose and prescribe and was therefore considered strictly unethical. These self-imposed limits on professional activity not only restricted the pharmacist's patient-care interventions to superficial encounters, but reinforced the widely accepted product-centered practice standard.

## Shifting professional values in pharmacy practice

In the 1930s, American pharmacy had described its passive relationship with physicians with such trite phrases as "the pharmacist is the handmaiden of the physician." As self-proclaimed "handmaidens," pharmacists viewed their service commitment to the physician as restricted solely to the accurate compounding of unquestioned prescription orders. While pharmacists envisioned themselves as stalwartly protecting the public from harm, ever alert for the occasional physician prescribing error, most felt uncomfortable discussing drug therapy with prescribers, content to discharge their professional duty at the distributive level only. Pharmacists felt obliged to seek prescribers' permission to clarify dosage directions or even add auxiliary labels; many pharmacists felt secure behind this self-imposed "ethical" barrier.

At about the same time, progressive pharmacy educators sought to introduce not only newer curricular materials based on the emerging pharmaceutical sciences of physical pharmacy and pharmacology, but also hoped to add a so-called "clinical" component to the pharmacist's education, a goal deferred to another generation of practitioner-educators nearly two decades later.[4] The pharmacists prepared by these "new" curricula were now expected to take advantage of commercially available products; moreover, they were also prepared to apply the principles of the new pharmaceutical sciences to their traditional compounding function. Educators felt that these new science-based pharmacists—who now could prepare sterile, isotonic ophthalmic solutions, create ointments and creams with enhanced percutaneous absorptive qualities, and discuss the kinetics of drug degradation with ease and authority— would finally emerge as respected members of the health-care team.[5]

By the 1960s, the growing preoccupation with profits in both hospital and community pharmacy settings had overshadowed and in many cases undermined the traditional service values associated with professional pharmacy practice. In hospitals, specialized pharmacy practitioners managed an increasingly efficient and complex drug distribution system, characterized by unit-dose systems and highly trained pharmacy technicians, and had as their goal providing "the right drug in the right dose to the right patient at the right time." In independent and chain pharmacies alike, many pharmacists retreated behind their prescription counters and concentrated on increasing their productivity and profits, continuing to treat their patients as mere customers. Others, like the visionary Eugene V. White, saw salvation in the "pharmaceutical center" concept, an office practice of pharmacy that promised to separate professional services from the commercialized atmosphere that had stultified pharmacy practice. White abandoned the unrelenting, profit-centered service value that characterized much of pharmacy practice, and adopted a more professional, patient-centered service value, one that utilized patient prescription records and stressed the interpersonal relationship between pharmacists and their patients.[6] While successful in carefully selected locations, the pharmaceutical center concept was far beyond the standard of American pharmacy practice and languished until incorporated into the clinically oriented practices typified by health maintenance organizations (HMOs) and neighborhood health centers nearly two decades later. Nevertheless, White's emphasis upon a patient-care value in pharmacy practice made a strong and lasting impression on practitioners across the nation, one that helped stimulate a transformation of the value system of the profession itself.

By the mid-1970s, however, evolving pharmacy practice and education began to be redefined in terms of a "clinically oriented" practice value that focussed on pharmacists providing effective drug therapy for their patients through extended interpersonal relationships. New drug regimens increased in complexity, generating such related professional challenges as drug interactions, drug product selection, and therapeutic drug interchanges, suggesting new professional roles and relationships for pharmacists. New, sophisticated dosage forms, such as transdermal patches and intraocular inserts, required not only extended professional knowledge on the part of the pharmacist, but the ability to explain their use to an often-puzzled patient. In hospital settings, pharmacy services expanded to include patient-care activities traditionally provided by nurses, such as intravenous admixture and medication administration programs. These new "clinical pharmacists" began to share the patient-centered value system of American medicine, abandoning subservience for collegiality while seeking—and to a certain extent achieving—professional parity with physicians. For their part, pharmacy educators responded by producing a new generation of scientifically sophisticated, clinically oriented practitioners through specialized "Doctor of Pharmacy" programs. Thus, just as pharmacists shifted the focus of their relationships with patients away from product-centered values, they also shifted the focus of their interprofessional relationships toward a patient-centered value system.

These shifts in professional values among pharmacists signaled the need for a deeper understanding of the human values associated with the patient-centered approach to professional pharmacy practice. Today, despite threatened reductions in patient services due to cost-containment initiatives in the health-care system, we appear to be witnessing a resurgence of the primacy of human values not only in medical and pharmacy practice, but throughout all health-care professions. This patient-sensitive professional attitude is reflected by an increased level of individualized professional service to both patients and physicians, and an increased emphasis upon the noneconomic values associated with drug therapy.

## Incorporating human values into pharmacy practice

Up to this point, we have concentrated upon pharmacy's reaction to the many changes that redefined the American health-care system during the past half-century. To what extent has this been a societal-driven phenomenon? Certainly, the American public has held its health-care practitioners to a legally defined standard of practice ever since these standards were promulgated in licensure laws. The information and technological explosions of the last thirty years led some public officials to question whether the minimalistic legal standards of practice were adequate to protect the public health, resulting in such societal interventions as mandatory continued professional education and periodic relicensure procedures designed to presumably safeguard the public from poorly informed or even incompetent health-care practitioners. This concern with professional competence, coupled with the consumerism movement of the 1970s, which demanded full disclosure of product and service information, higher standards of product safety, and fair and equitable health-care costs, all contributed to a publicly driven agenda for health-care professionals that seemed to demand ever-higher standards of professional practice.

**Recommitment to the human dignity of the individual.**  As health-care patterns became more complex and increasingly driven by cost-containment initiatives, some health-care practitioners began distancing themselves from their patients in the interest of efficiency: physicians felt they no longer could afford to make house calls, while nurses sought paraprofessional help for some traditional—if unpleasant—patient-care duties. Patients now found themselves numbered, counted, poked, prodded, and otherwise processed by the efficient, coldly clinical system of modern medical practice. The consumerism movement that had successfully demanded accountability from its health-care practitioners and struck down most of the so-called "ethical" bans on advertising of professional services now turned its attention to patient rights. The American Hospital Association, in response, quickly drafted a a statement on a "Patient's Bill of Rights," conferring upon beleaguered, processed patients the "rights" they already possessed, such as the "right" to be treated in a humane fashion or the "right" to examine their hospital bills. Patients and public officials alike soon saw through this transparent public relations façade, and sought real changes in the way patients were being treated.[7] In recent years, the effort to develop a broadly based patient's bill of rights has been elevated to the halls of our nation's Congress.

Pharmacists, who had once erected high, elevated prescription counters to screen themselves from direct, "inefficient" patient contact, responded by lowering these physical barriers, altering long-standing psychic constraints to good pharmacy practice. Pharmacists could now discuss complicated drug regimens and potentially embarrassing administration techniques privately with their patients rather than whispering sensitive directions *sotto voce* over a high prescription counter. Other pharmacists, now unfettered by outmoded, paternalistic ethical constraints enjoining them from discussing drug therapy with their patients, constructed patient consultation booths and restructured their entire practice to allow them to focus more intensely upon the pharmacist-patient encounter, creating a patient-centered, rather than a product-centered practice environment. Today, most health-care practitioners have replaced their earlier shrill public relations pronouncements with a sincere rededication to the primacy of human dignity in patient care.

**Shifting trends in disease and drug therapy.** The revolution in health-care values did not take place in a therapeutic vacuum. Indeed, such changes could not have occurred two generations ago. By the early 1950s, modern medicine had controlled most acute infectious diseases, and shifted its attention to treating the chronic, debilitating illnesses that infectious diseases had overshadowed by their sheer pervasiveness. Infant mortality receded, patients lived longer, more productive lives, maintained primarily by a host of sophisticated therapeutic agents. In the early 1960s, new psychotropic drugs controlled even acute mental disturbances, promising to empty mental institutions just as improved public health programs and streptomycin had emptied tuberculosis sanatoriums a decade earlier.[8] As a result, patients whose conditions would have warranted hospitalization or institutionalization a generation ago are now being treated by pharmacists on an out-patient basis. Other pharmacists extend the bounds of their practice to include supervising therapies, administering parenteral products in patients' homes, or coordinating hospice care. Moreover, drugs which were once available only by prescription are now available to an increasingly sophisticated public for uncontrolled autotherapy. As a result, pharmacists today deal more frequently with seriously ill or debilitated patients who require not only their full measure of professional expertise, but also an equally full measure of compassion and other human values from their health-care practitioners.

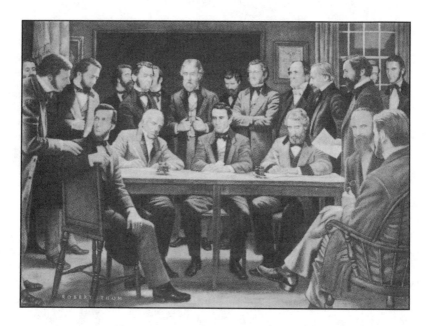

This painting by Robert Thom from the Great Moments in Pharmacy Series depicts the founding of the American Pharmaceutical Association in 1852. The Association established the first national code for pharmacists (see pp. 193-94). (*Illustration courtesy of Parke-Davis, division of Warner Lambert.*)

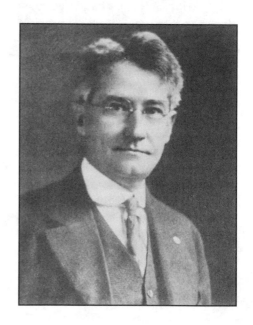

Charles H. LaWall (1871-1937), Dean of the Philadelphia College of Pharmacy (1918-37) and President of the American Pharmaceutical Association (1918-19), architect of the first modern code of ethics for American pharmacy (1922). (*Kremers Reference Files, F. B. Power Pharmaceutical Library, University of Wisconsin-Madison.*)

**Effective drug therapy as an expectation.** The past half-century has witnessed a meteoric, almost magical, transformation in drug therapy from palliative, symptomatic remedies to specific, highly potent agents. Once patients began to realize that the drugs prescribed by their physicians could actually eradicate their diseases, often with spectacular speed and efficacy, the miracle of modern medicine became not only a reality, but a common expectation. Just as modern surgical techniques have encouraged patients to elect cosmetic procedures once reserved for correcting serious facial deformities, so, too, have recent pharmacological advances encouraged patients to seek therapeutic treatment for such comparatively minor ailments as acne, hair loss, insomnia, or nervousness. Devotees of this new "pharmacological hedonism" translate ability to expectation; if a drug can produce a beneficial effect, it should be used without reservation, and at the patient's request, a situation further complicated by some pharmaceutical manufacturers' recent forays into direct-to-consumer advertising. Moreover, the aura once surrounding the so-called "miracle drugs" has been extended by the public to include all pharmacological categories; in the world of miracles, there is little margin for therapeutic failure or even compromise. Many patients view even minor side effects as unacceptable, and an ineffective drug regimen raises the specter of a malpractice suit. Such unrealistic public expectations place tremendous pressure on today's practicing physicians and pharmacists who must balance legitimate claims on their services with requests for mundane or even frivolous procedures or medications.


**Increasing consumer sophistication.** Leaders in organized medicine and pharmacy are keenly aware of the far-reaching impact that increased consumer knowledge and sophistication has had on their patients. While neither profession would willingly return to a standard of practice characterized by hastily scrawled Latinized prescriptions for mysterious medicines, few practitioners feel completely comfortable with patients who maintain their own personal laboratory values and vital signs, and ask for drugs by generic name, as supplied by the *Physicians' Desk Reference*. Fewer still would agree that fully informed patients can or should be full partners in establishing their own unique treatment plan, including their drug therapy.

Informed, medically sophisticated patients naturally seek to use their knowledge, and, in a sense, take control of their disease management and therapy. To an increasing extent, these patients expect their physicians and pharmacists to include them in many decisions regarding their therapy, rather than meekly submitting to the judgments of these practitioners. In recent years, this shift toward self-determination for one's personal health has been complicated by the wide range of alternative medicines which patients choose to complement their professionally managed therapy. Ideally, the physician, pharmacist, and patient should form a treatment team in which all participate to achieve an agreed-upon treatment goal. This emerging standard of practice, incorporated in the concept of pharmaceutical care, suggests that the pharmacist's responsibility now extends far beyond merely conveying the physician's instructions to the patient in a clear, concise manner. Rather, this standard expects pharmacists not only to help patients interpret their physicians' recommendations, but also to assist physicians in designing therapeutic treatment plans that both recognize enhanced patient knowledge and reflect a new respect for patient autonomy.

Unfortunately, not all patients have a full knowledge of their medical condition. Assuming all patients have such knowledge can lull practitioners into a false sense of security, leading them to take shortcuts in explaining directions for drug regimens, sometimes with tragic results. For example, during a routine follow-up examination, a woman who had been taking a powerful antihypertensive medication was told by her physician that her high blood pressure had been brought under control; unfortunately, he did not tell her that she must continue taking her medicine. Believing that the drug had done its work, the woman stopped taking her blood-pressure medication but did not notify her pharmacist who did not catch the change in her drug therapy; shortly thereafter, she suffered a crippling stroke. Both the physician and the pharmacist had overestimated the level of the woman's medical knowledge; neither had recognized the need to reinforce her understanding of her disease process and the necessity of continuing her drug therapy.

Despite such inherent communication difficulties created by the fragmented nature of our contemporary health-care system, today's pharmacists have a professional responsibility to assess the extent and depth of their patients' knowledge. Such assessments provide a solid base for pharmacists to establish the level of professional counseling their patients may require to successfully manage their drug therapy. Assisting patients to become legitimate partners in designing and managing their personal health-care plan without being perceived as either condescending or paternalistic emerges as one of pharmacy's most daunting professional challenges.

## The Pharmacist as a Health-Care Provider

Despite the potential conflicts that can occur between the traditional professional values of pharmacists and the changing societal expectations for medical and pharmacy practitioners outlined above, the pharmacist has recently begun to emerge not only as an active participant in the management of drug therapy, but also as a primary health-care provider. This transformation was slow and tortuous, however, constrained by narrowly conceived—and largely self-imposed—boundaries of practice. These traditional practice boundaries, both professional and legal in nature, are pervasive and continue to persist, hampering the professional development of the pharmacist as a full partner in the contemporary health-care system.

### Traditional boundaries of practice

Until comparatively recent times, a pharmacist's practice was bounded quite literally by the prescription counter. Behind the prescription counter, pharmacists compounded or otherwise prepared drugs for distribution in a secluded area, out of public view. At the prescription counter, pharmacists responded politely to requests for information from their patients, generally by simply reiterating the physician's instructions. It was unseemly for patients to know too much about the medicines their physicians prescribed, pharmacists argued. Pharmacists also responded to physicians' queries, but were careful not to stray beyond the rather shallow product information provided in manufacturers' catalogs or the package labeling. To patients and physicians alike, the pharmacist's counseling activities focussed on the drug product, not the therapy the drug was to provide.

**Technical competence in compounding and dispensing.** Mid-nineteenth-century American pharmacists saw incompetent, poorly educated practitioners as the greatest threat to their recognition as respected members of the health professions.[9] To that end, they organized state boards of pharmacy that served to measure at least the entry-level competence of potential practitioners and exclude the patently incompetent or the charlatan. To a large extent, these measurements relied upon board members' judgments of applicants' technical competence to compound prescription orders in an accurate and elegant manner. In a sense, these measurements came to define the practice of pharmacy itself. Despite higher educational standards and the increasing availability of commercially prepared pharmaceuticals, compounding and dispensing—and, later, dispensing itself—persisted as the *raison d'être* of both pharmacy education and practice well into the 1950s. Pharmacy curricula culminated in a series of courses titled "Dispensing," and state pharmacy practice acts defined the practice of pharmacy in terms of the compounding and dispensing function.[10] Those few pharmacists who sought expanded professional horizons were either ridiculed as impractical dreamers or chastised for trespassing upon the sacred domain of medicine. "Physicians diagnose and prescribe," the conventional wisdom reminded ambitious practitioners, "pharmacists dispense."

**Limited counseling and triage function.** Given the rigidly defined boundaries of professional practice described above, American pharmacists in the 1920s limited their "counseling" activities to recommending patent medicines and providing homely first-aid advice for life's aches and pains, minor injuries, and other annoyances. In the arena of prescription medication, traditional practice boundaries and contemporary codes of ethics strictly enjoined pharmacists from divulging any more information than provided by the physician's prescribed instructions.[11]

As modern and effective chemotherapeutic agents emerged in the 1940s, the therapeutic gulf between over-the-counter and prescribed medications grew wider and more distinct. Nevertheless, either silence or perfunctory, largely noninformative advice persisted as a standard of counseling practice among pharmacists throughout the 1960s.[12] When confronted by patients with direct requests for assistance with an alarming rash or another potentially serious ailment, most pharmacists satisfied themselves that they were performing an important and professional "triage function" by deciding which of their patients required medical attention by a physician and which could be satisfied by recommending an over-the-counter drug or another simple treatment plan.

## Legal boundaries of practice

For nearly 150 years, American pharmacy practice has been bounded and, in a sense, shaped by legislation. First through state laws restricting the sale of poisons, then through federal laws controlling the distribution of narcotics, pharmacists became accustomed to adhering to a wide range of regulations and legislation controlling their professional practice. Later, as therapeutic agents became more powerful and potentially more dangerous, some pharmacists actively sought the protection of both state and federal law and the resulting comfort afforded by a practice whose boundaries were defined by laws, rules, and regulations rather than by individual professional decisions. By the 1950s, this welter of federal and state legislation had removed all but a few vestigial traces of the professional discretion an earlier generation of pharmacists had enjoyed.

**Boundaries established by pharmacy practice acts.**    The early state pharmacy practice acts defined which drugs could be sold directly to the public, by whom, and under what conditions. These state acts primarily focussed upon the drug product itself and the manner in which it could be dispensed rather than any professional or consultative service the pharmacist could provide. In lieu of any federal legislation distinguishing between drug products that required a physician's supervision and those that could be safely used by the public for self-treatment, these early state pharmacy practice acts set aside the most potentially dangerous drugs in the pharmacist's armamentarium—poisons, narcotics, barbiturates, and hormones—for the physician's prescription, foreshadowing the rigorous prescription-only federal legislation of the 1950s.

Nevertheless, while strictly prohibited from diagnosing disease, prescribing drugs, or otherwise engaging in the practice of medicine, some pharmacists routinely engaged in recommending to their patients some of the more potent medicines available to them at that time. This practice of so-called "counter-prescribing" was savagely denounced by the medical profession, and stands in sharp contrast to the clearly defined standard of practice employed when these same drugs were dispensed on a physician's prescription: as we have suggested, pharmacists maintained a respectful silence when these drugs were prescribed, a silence sharply defined and undergirded by a professional code of ethics, but often offered free advice about their over-the-counter cousins.

**Boundaries established by state and federal agencies.**    While turn-of-the-century state pharmacy practice acts provided adequate controls over pharmacists and their distributive practices, these acts did not address the perplexing problems of drug adulteration and misbranding which had plagued generations of pharmacists. The Food and Drugs Act of 1906 brought both domestic manufacturers of legitimate, so-called "ethical" pharmaceuticals[13] and patent medicines and nostrums under the umbrella of federal legislation for the first time. The Act not only effectively eliminated adulterated drugs, but also controlled misbranding by establishing stringent labeling requirements. Pharmaceutical manufacturers were required to identify the names and amounts of the active ingredients in their products and label them with honest therapeutic claims.[14] Some manufacturers proudly met the new federal mandate, changing their formulas or dropping label claims that could not be sustained in court;[15] others evaded the law by simply transferring false or misleading label claims to their advertising.

By the late 1930s, as therapeutic agents became more powerful—and potentially more dangerous—the federal government looked to pharmaceutical manufacturers to establish stricter guidelines to better distinguish between drugs that needed some medical supervision and those that could be used safely for self-treatment by the general public, a function primarily controlled by state pharmacy laws. It soon became clear, however, that America's pharmaceutical manufacturers held a wide spectrum of values when it came to distinguishing between drugs for which prescriptions were recommended and their over-the-counter cousins: Some of these manufacturers, seeking a broader market for their drug products, developed complicated—if strictly legal—labeling for products that had traditionally been distributed under medical supervision; other manufacturers, wary of the legal liability associated with injuries caused by unsupervised drug use or interested in exploiting the more exclusive prescription-only cachet for their drug products, developed overly restrictive labeling for products that had traditionally been sold at the corner drugstore.

Prompted by the tragedy of the Elixir of Sulfanilamide poisonings and the ensuing public furor,[16] the federal Food, Drug and Cosmetic Act of 1938 required pharmaceutical manufacturers of new drug products to document that their products could be safely used before marketing them. The Act not only addressed purity and safety, but subtly affected labeling requirements as well. Manufacturers were required to develop "adequate directions for use," later defined as directions a lay person could understand well enough to use a drug product safely. Drugs labeled "Caution: to be used only by or on the prescription of a physician, dentist, or veterinarian," however, were exempted from bearing such directions, a provision that had the unintended effect of encouraging many pharmaceutical manufacturers to designate all their products for prescription use only. Some manufacturers labeled a drug product with "adequate directions for use"; others labeled the same drug product with the "Caution:" statement; some did both.

The resulting confusion posed both a legal quagmire and a potential professional dilemma to practicing pharmacists: drugs not covered by state board regulations, such as sulfonamides and penicillin, could be legally distributed by the pharmacist without a prescription. The "Caution:" statement was a warning statement to the patient; it did not prohibit the sale of a certain class of drug products. Pharmacists either filled prescriptions for these products or solicitously inquired if their patients were under a doctor's care before dispensing the products. Less scrupulous pharmacists who sold products without such assurances were subject to federal prosecution, not because they had dispensed a "Caution:" drug without a prescription, but because they had caused the drug to be "misbranded," that is, dispensed without "adequate directions for use."[17] The resulting confusion and specter of increased legal liability frustrated and worried even the most conscientious pharmacist.

In 1948, Congress passed the Miller Amendment to the 1938 Act, extending the definition of interstate commerce of drug products to include all levels of distribution from manufacturer to consumer, including the pharmacists' final repackaging and labeling activities. By 1950, the situation had become critical: Pharmacists prosecuted under the new law sought assistance from their professional associations; organized pharmacy, in turn, sought a legal clarification of the matter. The Durham-Humphrey Amendment of 1951 supplied the long-needed definition of the kinds of drugs that must be labeled for prescription use only.[18] Moreover, the Amendment prohibited prescription refills without the expressed authorization of the prescriber, eliminating the time-honored professional prerogative of the pharmacist to monitor and control their patients' drug therapy, thereby substituting federal law for a traditional ethic of the profession. Hailed at its passage as a sensible solution to a vexing professional problem, the Durham-Humphrey Amendment is now often criticized for not only eliminating traditional professional functions, but also for seriously hampering the pharmacist's professional development as a full partner with the physician in today's emerging health-care environment.[19]

The Amendment had profound ethical and legal ramifications for American pharmacy practice. In the arena of ethics, the Amendment replaced the pharmacist's traditional duty to warn patients of the potential dangers which might be associated with continuing their prescription drug therapy with a simple legal rule: prescriptions could be refilled only by a physician's authorization. Moreover, by providing a legal—rather than a professional—basis for deciding whether or not to refill patients' prescriptions, the Amendment had the unintended effect of subtly shifting the nature of pharmacists' legal liability, as reflected by the spate of malpractice claims during the past decade.[20]

**Boundaries established by case law.** During the decades following World War II, the American public became accustomed to the therapeutic miracles it received in prescription bottles. Antiinfectives, tranquilizers, and, later, oral contraceptives were cursorily provided by harried pharmacists increasingly preoccupied with managing a rapidly increasing prescription volume, rising overhead costs, and ruinous price-cutting battles. These new drugs were not only more potent, but possessed a much narrower range of therapeutic safety; there was little, if any, room for error. Pharmacists soon learned they could no longer solely rely upon their memories or notes scribbled upon the back of prescription orders to alert them to the new professional challenge of drug-drug interactions. Pharmacists employed crude handwritten patient prescription profiles to detect drug interactions, an innovation heralded as an opportunity for an expanded professional function, a function that soon became ingrained as a new standard of practice. This new standard soon became viewed as a legal standard of practice as well: Pharmacists were now expected to detect and warn their patients of potential drug interactions and to intervene with the physician to avoid therapeutic misadventures; pharmacists who did not employ these new drug monitoring systems faced the very real risk of being considered professionally irresponsible or, worse, being convicted of malpractice for disregarding their new legal duty to warn. This new legal responsibility, combined with the public's concern for professional accountability, and fanned by the consumerism movement of the 1960s, increased the professional liability of the practicing pharmacist to a level undreamed of a decade earlier. In an increasing litigious society, patients sued their pharmacist if they felt they had been injured, treated unfairly, or just slighted. Pharmacy malpractice insurance premiums soared, and pharmacists became acutely aware of their expanded legal liability. This shift in the nature of professional liability, therefore, has altered the very nature of contemporary courtroom cases affecting pharmacists by emphasizing the importance of pharmacists' duty to warn rather than their failure to follow federal and state drug law. This specter of increased professional liability has thus profoundly affected pharmacists' view of the importance of performing their professional functions.

## Expanding boundaries of practice

By the early 1950s, Americans had stopped worrying about the threatened postwar recession; the United States economy was booming: families moved to the rapidly expanding suburbs to enjoy a lifestyle formerly reserved for the affluent; American pharmacy enjoyed unprecedented growth, particularly in the rapidly developing drugstore chain sector, a growth accompanied by fierce competition. America's pharmaceutical manufacturers embarked upon expanded programs of research and development, filling the drug market with new and more effective trademarked prescription specialties, heavily advertised in medical journals and promoted by an aggressive sales force. Between 1948 and 1960, for example, a period of relatively slow population growth, the number of prescriptions dispensed increased by 70 per cent, yet accounted for nearly a four-fold increase in prescription dollar volume.[21] What Americans wanted most, community pharmacists decided, were large, modern, self-service stores, quick service, and low prices; hospital pharmacists responded by developing drug delivery systems characterized by accuracy, efficiency, and economy.

Expanding societal expectations. The consumerism movement of the early 1970s focussed the American public's attention upon professional accountability, both in terms of competency to practice, which resulted in legislation mandating continued professional education, and in terms of enhanced standards of practice, which were debated extensively by the pharmaceutical community throughout the decade and finally set down on paper in 1979.[22] Patients challenged physicians and pharmacists alike with their demands to become active, knowledgeable partners in the design of their drug therapy. The *Physicians' Desk Reference*, once restricted to professional distribution, became a best-seller at America's bookstores. Activists petitioned legislators to strike down laws and state board regulations prohibiting prescription drug advertising and generic drug substitution, while the profession itself responded with such remedies as prescription price posting, patient prescription profiles, and patient counseling in the community setting, and instituted drug utilization review and drug formularies in the hospital setting.[23] These public and professional initiatives focussed upon patient care, first as a concept, then as a right. Practitioners began to realize that they could not provide individualized patient care without caring for patients as individuals.

At the same time, public health activists, including some of the more visionary members of the health professions, expanded the concept of health beyond the mere absence of disease, envisioning a new high plain of personal health, which they termed "high-level wellness." Concerned and determined pharmacists increased their health promotions, adding blood-pressure monitoring devices to their pharmacies, providing diabetes screening programs, or offering cholesterol-level determinations to their patrons.

**Evolving professional functions.** By the 1960s, compounding had become a scientifically based, highly technical, and sophisticated function, but one rarely performed in practice, a mere remnant of a proud professional past. Dispensing itself was recognized and institutionalized as the legitimate and sole professional function of the pharmacist. Isolated from all other aspects of patient care, the pharmacist's professional function typically ended once the prescription was brought to the prescription counter or delivered to the hospital ward. Dissatisfied by the lack of challenge and prestige associated with the dispensing function, some pharmacists sought to expand their diminishing professional role by engaging in other product-related professional activities: Some sought expanded professional prestige by promoting themselves as advisors to the physician, comparing and contrasting commercially available drug products; others found solace in advising the public on the use of nonprescription medication or durable medical equipment; still others established patient prescription record systems as an efficient way to locate prescriptions and prepare tax records.

In the 1970s, pharmacists continued to develop other product-related professional services appropriate to their science-based education: To some educators and practitioners, the rapidly expanding availability of generic drug products and the subsequent repeal of the so-called "antisubstitution laws" signaled the need for an expanded advisory role to physicians in the area of drug product selection, particularly in institutional settings, where pharmacists now participated in the deliberations of pharmacy and therapeutics committees. Some pharmacists studied charts allowing them to compare and contrast nonprescription drug products; others urged Congress to establish a third class of drugs which could be sold only by a pharmacist;[24] still others modified patient prescription record systems to serve as the basis for detecting drug interactions or potential abuse problems. The development of computerized patient prescription record systems, with sophisticated drug interaction modules, however, transformed the pharmacist's informational function from the mere collecting, retrieving, and transmitting of data to the actual interpretation of clinically significant interactions, a role for which many pharmacists were ill-prepared. Similarly, it soon became clear that pharmacists could not be expected to interpret or even have access to the welter of chemical, pharmaceutical—and later biological—equivalency data necessary to effectively help the physician select drug products. At the same time, a new breed of clinical pharmacists argued persuasively that professional redemption lay in a radical shift from a product-oriented to a patient-oriented practice, a practice that emphasized expanded patient counseling and, in a sense, a return to patient-care functions reminiscent of an earlier generation of pharmacy practitioners.

**The concept of pharmaceutical care.** In a seminal paper titled "Opportunities and Responsibilities in Pharmaceutical Care," C. Douglas Hepler and Linda M. Strand proposed a new philosophy of pharmacy practice far beyond the rather limited expectations of most pharmacy practitioners, even those dedicated to the patient-oriented practices embraced by the term "clinical pharmacy." Speaking at a 1989 conference focussing on evolving pharmacy practice for the twenty-first century, Hepler and Strand reviewed the alarming extent of drug-related morbidity and mortality in the American health-care system. They concluded that this problem could only be addressed by a fundamental change in the pharmacist's professional function, a concept they referred to as "pharmaceutical care."

Defining pharmaceutical care as "the responsible provision of drug therapy for the purpose of achieving definite outcomes that improve a patient's quality of life," Hepler and Strand argued that the costly social problem of "drug misadventuring" could be reduced or even eliminated by pharmacists' intervention. Rather than restricting the pharmacist's professional role to merely supplying and monitoring drug therapy, Hepler and Strand built upon concepts of clinical pharmacy to create "a process in which a pharmacist cooperates with a patient and other health professionals in designing, implementing, and monitoring a therapeutic plan that will produce specific therapeutic outcomes for the patient." Central to their shared vision is the establishment of a "mutually beneficial

exchange in which the patient grants authority to the provider, and
the provider gives competence and commitment to the patient."[25]

Leaders in the generally conservative world of pharmaceutical education embraced the philosophy of pharmaceutical care
with an ardor rarely seen in academic circles. The American Association of Colleges of Pharmacy's Commission to Implement
Change in Pharmaceutical Education hailed the new philosophy as
"truly a revolutionary concept in the practice of pharmacy" not
only because its practitioners assume responsibility for the outcomes of drug therapy in patients, but because "it espouses CARING,
an emotional commitment to the welfare of patients as individuals
who require and deserve pharmacists' compassion, concern and
trust." While some skeptics dismissed the Commission's enthusiasm as yet another attempt to justify the expansion of the clinical
component of the pharmacy curriculum, they could not ignore the
Commission's recommendations that the Association "adopt pharmaceutical care as the philosophy of pharmacy practice on which
practitioner education must be based" and that member colleges
and faculty "immediately commit themselves to curricular changes
which . . . engenders competencies and outcomes essential to pharmaceutical care," both of which were adopted by the Association's
House of Delegates in 1992.[26] That same year, the Association
voted to support the inclusion of these outcomes and competencies
in the revised accreditation standards of the American Council on
Pharmaceutical Education, the body which accredits all entry-level
pharmaceutical education programs.[27]

## Concluding Remarks

The practice philosophy of pharmaceutical care has acquired an
enviable currency in the world of pharmaceutical education and
the world of pharmacy practice as well. When fully implemented,
the philosophy will achieve the redefinition of professional pharmacy practice functions that its proponents envision. To be sure,
the profession faces daunting challenges to its traditional functional autonomy: state and federal governments, insurance companies, and other third parties exert unrelenting pressures for cost
control and enhanced professional service in the delivery of prescription and nonprescription medication to the public. The profession has responded to these pressures by increasingly relying on
paraprofessional help, robotics, and computer-assisted patient in-

formation systems to manage its interpersonal patient-care functions. Just as pharmacy has learned it can no longer focus exclusively upon the mere safe distribution of drugs or even upon expanded clinical functions in order to justify its societal function, it may also learn it cannot solely rely upon the enhanced, personalized clinical services encompassed by the concept of pharmaceutical care for its *raison d'être*.

As desirable as these sophisticated distributive and enhanced clinical services may be, they cannot substitute for the value-based professional decisions that are the hallmark of a profession. Such values as compassion, faithfulness, and fairness define the very essence of pharmaceutical care; as this concept matures, practitioners will identify other associated virtues and values. By not reflecting upon the human values associated with pharmacy as a practice, pharmacists may weaken the fundamental moral underpinnings of pharmacy as a profession. Pharmaceutical care in its fullest sense involves professional care decisions beyond enhanced therapeutic outcomes. Practitioners who embrace the tenets of pharmaceutical care would do well to consider the moral and ethical implications implicit within this new philosophy of practice. It is these implications and the moral and ethical basis for the professional practice of pharmacy that we will be examining in the ensuing chapters.

## Study Questions

1.1 Express, in your own words, the moral basis for the profession of pharmacy.

1.2 Explain and defend the personal value(s) that you consider the most important to the ethical practice of pharmacy.

1.3 Outline the implications for expanded ethical responsibilities for pharmacy practitioners as they embrace the tenets of pharmaceutical care.

1.4 What is the most compelling moral aspect of making a commitment to the welfare of patients based upon compassion, concern, and trust?

# References

1.  U.S.P. and N.F. "propaganda" was one of the activities undertaken by the American Pharmaceutical Association's new local branches in 1906, when these compendia became the federally recognized standards for American drug products. By the late 1930s, pharmacists' interest in physicians writing individualized prescriptions for their patients—rather than prescribing standardized commercial products—prompted the Association to organize a series of conferences on the topic. See C. S. N. Hallberg, "The American Pharmaceutical Association—The Post-Graduate Course for the Retail Pharmacist," *Bulletin of the American Pharmaceutical Association 1*:10 (October, 1906), p. 314; "Meeting of the State Committees on U.S.P. and N.F. Promotion," *Journal of the American Pharmaceutical Association 27*:11 (November, 1938), pp. 1161-62; and "Conference of State Committees on U.S.P.-N.F. Promotion," *ibid. 28*:11 (November, 1939), pp. 943-44.

2.  Pharmacy historian Glenn Sonnedecker notes that minimum standards for hospital pharmacists, adopted by the American College of Surgeons in 1936, and the emergence of the American Society of Hospital Pharmacists in 1942 as an independent organization signaled new stature and goals for the specialty. "What could scarcely be foreseen was the transformation that would occur within a quarter century to bring the hospital pharmacist out of his basement 'drug room' and into an unprecedented professional enthusiasm and stature in the history of American pharmacy." Glenn Sonnedecker, *Kremers and Urdang's History of Pharmacy*, 4th ed., rev. (Philadelphia: J. B. Lippincott Company, 1976), p. 320.

3.  Sonnedecker notes that "grossly commercialized" conditions of practice, where prescription service was "exploited through flamboyant advertising" became widespread during the 1950s, "bringing pressure especially on urban pharmacists who tried to maintain full professional services and the standards that have given pharmacy its standing as one of the health professions." *Ibid.*, p. 297.

4.  In the early 1940s, for example, L. Wait Rising developed an experimental course in which students did "a great variety of laboratory work under actual conditions of practice with close supervision by both professional pharmacist and instructor." L. Wait Rising, "Theory and Practice Can Be Combined," *American Journal of Pharmaceutical Education 9*:4 (October, 1945), p. 558. Heber W. Youngken, Jr., later reported that the innovation created "a state of confusion . . . whereby similar programs in pharmaceutical education were . . . discouraged." H[eber] W. Youngken, Jr., "The Washington Experiment—Clinical Pharmacy," *American Journal of Pharmaceutical Education 17*:1 (January, 1953), p. 67.

5.  In 1974, for example, University of California School of Pharmacy Dean Jere E. Goyan remarked that these "new" curricula produced "a generation of pharmacists who knew the chemical structures of phenobarbital and procaine, including several pathways to their synthesis, and other arcane knowledge for which, to put it politely, they found little use." Jere E. Goyan, "Pharmacy Practice—Structure and Function,"

*American Journal of Pharmaceutical Education 38*:5 (December, 1974), p. 693.

6. "The primary element must be the personal, professional relationship between the pharmacist and his patient based on the sincere interest of the pharmacist in the health and welfare of his patient and his family," White stated in 1965. "I have found if you convince the patient his health and welfare is your objective and your intention is not a selfish mercenary one he will literally beat a path to your pharmacy door." Eugene V. White, "Behind the Scenes of the Pharmaceutical Center," *Journal of the American Pharmaceutical Association NS5*:10 (October, 1965), p. 532.

7. See, for example, "Statement on a Patient's Bill of Rights," in André L. Lee and Godfrey Jacobs, "Workshop Airs Patients' Rights," *Hospitals 47*:4 (February 16, 1973), p. 41. The statement was affirmed by the Board of Trustees of the American Hospital Association on November 17, 1972. Ethicist Willard Gaylin characterizes the Statement as "not only pretentious but deceptive" and charges that this document "perpetuates the very paternalism that precipitated the abuses" it seeks to correct. "It is the thief lecturing his victim on self-protection," Gaylin thunders. "It is not for the hospital community to outline the rights it will offer, but rather for the patient consumer to delineate and then demand those rights to which he feels entitled." Willard Gaylin, "The Patient's Bill of Rights," *Saturday Review of the Sciences 1*:2 February 24, 1973), p. 22. A revision of the Bill of Rights was approved by the American Hospital Association's Board of Trustees on October 21, 1992 (see Appendix B).

8. For the interplay between modern public health and antibiotic drug therapy in their treatment of tuberculosis, see James Bordley, III and A. McGehee Harvey, *Two Centuries of American Medicine, 1776-1976* (Philadelphia: W. B. Saunders Company, 1976), pp. 206-13 and 456-60.

9. Thus, in 1854 William Procter, Jr., and Edward Parrish complained bitterly about the nation's "incompetent drug clerks," most of whom were neither trained through a legally indentured apprenticeship nor held to an honor-bound obligation. "These clerks in turn become principals, and have the direction of others—alas! for the progeny that some of them bring forth, as ignorance multiplied by ignorance will produce neither knowledge nor skill." W[illiam] Procter, Jr., E[dward] Parrish, D[avid] Stewart, and J[ohn] Meakim, "Address to the Pharmaceutists of the United States," *Proceedings of the American Pharmaceutical Association 3* (1854), p. 14.

10. As late as 1960, for example, the AACP-NABP Joint Committee to Redefine the Term "Pharmacy" also redefined the "practice of pharmacy" in terms of the "important distributive function of the pharmacist" which "includes prescription drugs as well as those sold directly to the consumer," and hoped that the new definition would be incorporated into state pharmacy practice acts. See Linwood F. Tice, "Report of the AACP-NABP Joint Committee to Redefine the Term 'Pharmacy'," *American Journal of Pharmaceutical Education 25*:1 (Winter, 1961), p. 102.

11. The pharmacist "should never discuss the therapeutic effect of a Physician's prescription with a patron nor disclose details of composition which the Physician has withheld, suggesting to the patient that such details can be properly discussed with the prescriber only," the 1922 APhA Code intoned. See "Code of Ethics of the American Pharmaceutical Association," *Journal of the American Pharmaceutical Association*

*11*:9 (September, 1922), p. 729.
12. The 1952 APhA Code continued to enjoin the pharmacist to "not dis-
    cuss the therapeutic effects or composition of a prescription with a pa-
    tient. When such questions are asked, he suggests that the qualified
    practitioner is the proper person with whom such matters should be
    discussed." This restrictive prohibition was deleted from the 1969 ver-
    sion of the Code. See "Code of Ethics of the American Pharmaceutical
    Association," *Journal of the American Pharmaceutical Association 13*:10
    (October, 1952), p. 722; and "APhA Code of Ethics," *ibid. NS9*:11 (No-
    vember, 1969), p. 552.
13. The term "ethical specialty" was coined in 1876 by Detroit drug manu-
    facturer Frederick Stearns to distinguish his line of "simple prepara-
    tions in popular-sized packages, bearing full directions for use and . . . a
    plain statement of the names and quantities of their ingredients." See
    "Frederick Stearns, Pharmacist: An Appreciation," *The New Idea 27*:1
    (First Quarter, 1905), p. 3. The term "ethical" was later used to distin-
    guish manufactured drug products promoted to the medical profession
    from those promoted directly to the public.
14. For a brief, insightful historical development of the 1906 Act, see Wallace
    F. Janssen, "Pharmacy and the Food and Drug Law: A Significant Re-
    lationship," *American Pharmacy NS21*:4 (April, 1981), pp. 212-21. An
    earlier piece of federal legislation, the Import Drugs Act of 1848, pro-
    vided for laboratory inspections at ports of entry and for detention, de-
    struction, or re-exporting of shipments not meeting pharmacopeial stan-
    dards, but suffered from lack of enforcement. *Ibid.*, p. 214.
15. Thus, Lloyd Brothers, the Cincinnati-based manufacturer of single-in-
    gredient "Specific Medicines," remarked in their 1921 catalogue that
    "the fact that when the National law passed, every Specific Medicine
    was found to conform to its severest requirement, was a great satisfac-
    tion to physicians and a matter of pride to us. Every Specific Medicine
    in every jobbing house in America is correctly labeled in the form the
    Government approves, and is true to name and quality." Lloyd Broth-
    ers, *Dose Book of Fine Medicinal Specialties* (Lloyd Brothers: Cincin-
    nati, Ohio, 1921), pp. 66-67.
16. For example, Mrs. Maise Nidiffer, who had lost her six-year-old daugh-
    ter to the Elixir, wrote a heart-rendering letter to President Franklin D.
    Roosevelt. "It is my plea that you will take steps to prevent such sales
    of drugs that will take little lives and leave such suffering behind," Mrs.
    Nidiffer begged, adding, "Surely we can have laws governing doctors
    also who will give such a medicine, not knowing to what extent its dan-
    ger." H[enry] A. Wallace, "Report of the Secretary of Agriculture on
    Deaths Due to Elixir Sulfanilamide-Massengill," *Elixir Sulfanilamide:
    Letter from the Secretary of Agriculture Transmitting in Response to Sen-
    ate Resolution No. 194, a Report on Elixir Sulfanilamide-Massengill*, Sen-
    ate Document No. 124, 75th Congress, 2d Session (Washington, D.C.:
    Government Printing Office, 1937), p. 8.
17. Janssen, "Pharmacy and the Food and Drug Law," (n. 14) p. 218. "This
    legally complex approach was cumbersome, confusing and contradic-
    tory," Janssen contends. "Moreover, it was difficult for FDA . . . to en-
    force the new distinction between prescription and OTC drugs . . . [since]
    the law contained no definition of a prescription drug, and FDA had not
    presumed to provide one."

18. For a contemporary analysis of the Durham-Humphrey controversy, see Robert P. Fischelis, "The Pharmacist's Right and Duty to Exercise Professional Judgment," *Journal of the American Pharmaceutical Association* (Practical Pharmacy Edition) *11*:4 (April, 1950), pp. 218-25.

19. For the most part, American pharmacists have aggressively sought legislative protection, while at the same time bitterly decrying governmental intervention in their professional practice. Charles D. Hepler notes that the Durham-Humphrey amendment "prevented pharmacists from recommending many useful drugs and limited the scope of their judgment and problem-solving." Charles D. Hepler, "The Third Wave in Pharmaceutical Education: The Clinical Movement," *American Journal of Pharmaceutical Education 51*:4 (Winter, 1987), pp. 371-72.

20. See, for example, Jesse C. Vivian, "Pharmacy Malpractice: Crisis or Crucible?" *American Pharmacy NS34*:4 (April, 1994), pp. 25-30; and Walter L. Fitzgerald, Jr., "Legal Control of Pharmacy Services," in *OBRA '90: A Practical Guide to Effecting Pharmaceutical Care*, edited by Bruce R. Canaday (Washington, D.C.: American Pharmaceutical Association, 1994), pp. 47-55.

21. "Rx Sales Outstrip U.S. Income Growth," *Drug Topics 93*:9 (April 25, 1949), p. 1; and "Average Doctor Wrote 167 Fewer Rxs in 1960 Than In 1959, A.D. Study Shows," *American Druggist 144*:3 (August 7, 1961), p. 7; Pharmacy historian Glenn Sonnedecker attributes this growth to "therapeutically active substances being dispensed more often individually (rather than combined in a single prescription); to more effective medicaments becoming available, leading to their freer use and sometimes overuse; to a more affluent society in the period; growth of 'third-party payment'; and other factors." See Sonnedecker, *Kremers and Urdang's History of Pharmacy* (n. 2), p. 313; also see Pharmaceutical Manufacturers Association, *Prescription Drug Industry Fact Book* (Washington, D.C.: Pharmaceutical Manufacturers Association, [1973]), p. 31.

22. The new "Standards of Practice" for the profession of pharmacy were completed in 1979 after "six grueling years of work and an investment by the American Pharmaceutical Association and the American Association of Colleges of Pharmacy of more than $250,000." The Standards included sections on the general management and administration of the pharmacy, activities related to processing prescriptions, patient-care functions, and the education of health-care professionals and patients. See Samuel H. Kalman and John F. Schlegel, "Standards of Practice for the Profession of Pharmacy," *American Pharmacy NS19*:3 (March, 1979), pp. 133-45. Also see "National Study Shows What Pharmacists Actually Do," *ibid.*, pp. 146-47.

23. In the early 1970s, for example, the National Association of Retired Persons was active at the state level seeking repeal of antisubstitution laws, while Ralph Nader's consumer group Public Interest won a court battle allowing advertising of prescription prices. See Mickey C. Smith and David A. Knapp, *Pharmacy, Drugs and Medical Care*, 3rd ed. (Baltimore: Williams & Wilkins), p. 148.

24. As early as 1960, the American Pharmaceutical Association's Committee on Legislation drew the Association's attention to "an intermediate category of drugs which either were formerly under the prescription legend or which contain one or more drugs which by themselves are prescription legend drugs. All these drugs must have their distribution su-

pervised by registered pharmacists." See "Legal Blotter: Drug Classification Questions," *Journal of the American Pharmaceutical Association NS5*:1 (January, 1965), pp. 30-31. While never implemented, the concept became a *cause célèbre* for the Association throughout the 1960s. See, for example, Richard P. Penna, "Control of Over-the-Counter Medication," *ibid. NS5*:11 (November, 1965), pp. 584-86; Harold L. Marquis, "Problems Involved in Drug Reclassification," *ibid. NS7*:4 (April, 1967), pp. 170-73; and a characteristically forceful defense by Executive Director William S. Apple, "Pharmacy's New Rx Evolution," *ibid. NS7*:9 (September, 1967), pp. 474- 77, 484.

25. Charles D. Hepler and Linda M. Strand, "Opportunities and Responsibilities in Pharmaceutical Care," *American Journal of Pharmaceutical Education 53*:[5] (Winter Supplement, 1989), p. 15S.

26. Commission to Implement Change in Pharmaceutical Education, "Background Paper II: Entry Level, Curricular Outcomes, Curricular Content and Educational Process," *AACP News* Special Report (March, 1991), pp. 1 and 9.

27. Robert A. Sandmann, "Chair Report of the Bylaws and Policy Development Committee," *American Journal of Pharmaceutical Education 56*:[5] (Winter Supplement, 1992), p. 14S.

# Suggested Readings

Buerki, Robert A. "History and Human Values in Ethics Instruction." In *Teaching and Learning Strategies in Pharmacy Ethics*, edited by Amy M. Haddad. Omaha, Nebraska: Creighton University, 1992, pp. 43-52.

Hughes, Thomas F., and Eckel, Fred M. "Ethical Issues Associated with Managed Care Pharmacy Services." *Topics in Hospital Pharmacy Management 10*:3 (November, 1990), pp. 30-38.

LaWall, Charles H. "Pharmaceutical Ethics: A Historical Review of the Subject with Examples of Codes Adopted or Suggested at Different Periods, Together with a Suggested Code for Adoption by Present-Day Associations." *Journal of the American Pharmaceutical Association 10*:11 (November, 1921), pp. 895-910, and *ibid. 10*:12 (December, 1921), pp. 961-64.

McMahon, Thomas F. "The Professional's Responsibility." *Journal of the American Pharmaceutical Association NS12*:7 (July, 1972), pp. 358-59.

Veatch, Robert M. "Professional Prerogatives: Perspectives of an Ethicist." *American Journal of Pharmaceutical Education 55*:1 (Spring, 1991), pp. 74-78.

# CHAPTER 2

# FOUNDATIONS OF ETHICAL
# DECISION-MAKING

For centuries, pharmacists have sought to maintain ethical standards as an integral part of their emerging professional character. The recent shift toward a patient-centered practice of pharmacy has presented practitioners in all practice settings with a variety of new challenges. Expanded patient contacts have resulted in improved patient care, more rational drug therapy, and higher rates of compliance; however, these intensely personal, even intimate, contacts have increased the pharmacist's exposure to ethical and moral dilemmas as well. Moreover, the issues underlying these dilemmas tend to be more complex and significant than the product-centered problems faced by earlier generations of practitioners.

Unfortunately, too many pharmacists react emotionally to these perplexing ethical dilemmas or rely on their experience or instinct to solve problems as they arise, denying themselves the satisfying, often fulfilling, opportunity to engage in ethical reasoning. Ethical reasoning is a complex, learned process that involves sorting through a complex mélange of ethical principles, virtues and values, rules and codes. Furthermore, because each ethical encounter is as unique as the individuals involved, it is difficult for practitioners to generalize from one specific case to another. This uniqueness of ethical dilemmas encountered in practice requires pharmacists to repeat the process of ethical reasoning with each encounter. Moreover, since some specific actions or outcomes are more acceptable than others when solving ethical dilemmas, pharmacists must be able to explain their choices and defend their ethical decision-making. Resolving ethical conflicts through reflective ethical analysis can not only lead pharmacy practitioners to a greater sense of personal worthiness but may represent the most laudable form of professional behavior within their practice.

What are the agreed-upon personal values or ethical practice standards of American pharmacy as the profession enters the twenty-first century? Are the therapeutic misadventures Hepler and Strand hope to resolve in their call for pharmaceutical care based upon an "ethical mandate" or an "ethical imperative" or are these merely rhetorical, imprecise applications of the term "ethical?" Can we identify time-honored moral principles and widely recognized ethical theories that apply to all generations of pharmacists in every practice setting? Are there commonly identified virtues so associated with the practice of pharmacy that they are embodied in every "ethical" pharmacy practitioner? Are the ethical norms reflected in pharmacy's codes of ethics defined by a national body representing pharmacists, by pharmacy faculty in the classroom, by pharmacist-preceptors in the experiential program, or is ethical conduct merely what most pharmacists informally agree is "right" or "proper?"

## Ethical Theories and Principles as a Framework for Decision-Making

All persons, pharmacists included, draw upon a wide range of experiences and influences that converge to form their personal value system. The influences of our parents, friends, teachers, religious leaders, and others all combine to forge a basic value system that continues to expand during our years of professional pharmacy education and practical experience and into our professional practice. Our professional decisions flow from this unique, highly complex set of values we have acquired. How does our value system influence our professional decision-making in pharmacy practice?

If we highly value interpersonal relationships with our patients, we might make decisions that enhance these relationships, rather than those that may conform to a formal statement contained in a professional code of ethics. Some pharmacists, for example, may place great importance on *non*personal values, such as a strong allegiance to the bureaucracy embodied in the Medicaid program or any of the myriad of third-party prescription plan policies with which pharmacists contend on a daily basis. These pharmacists who value bureaucratic rules designed primarily for internal efficiency, rather than the values associated with good patient care, may refuse to continue maintenance therapy to an indigent patient because of certain third-party program constraints. "The structures of the institution have become so complex that it is difficult to know where and what the work of caring for the sick is, or ought to be," ethicist Albert Jonsen reflected recently. "Where in that vast complex of systems is . . . health care practiced?"[1]

Other pharmacists who value the altruism associated with good patient care may circumvent these rules or even risk loss of reimbursement for their professional services by providing this therapy. Still other pharmacists may hold competing values pulling them in opposite directions and make practice decisions based upon whim or instinct, the idiosyncrasies of certain patients, or even their appearance, resulting in inconsistent professional behavior. Regardless of the genesis or composition of their individual value systems, however, pharmacists must realize that their professional decisions are ultimately guided by their personal values. For this reason, we should closely examine and reaffirm the unique, personal set of values that form the basis for the ethical decisions we make in practice.

Scholars of ethics and social psychology have recently expanded their approach to traditional theories to include *social contracts* and the *ethics of care*. A social contract exists when two mutually dependent groups in a society recognize certain expectations of one another and conduct their affairs according to those expectations. As a health profession, pharmacy was brought into being in response to society's needs and expectations and continues to exist because of the mutual dependence between pharmacy and society at large.[2] Unlike legal contracts, which are precise and have implicit sanctions, social contracts are unwritten, leaving the specific duties and actions expected of health-care practitioners and their patients to a process of reasoning and discernment. At best, professional codes of ethics may offer the nearest thing to written obligations of the partners, providing action-guides in cases of ethical dilemmas.

The ethics of care, often associated with social psychologist Carol Gilligan, emphasizes ethical actions rooted in a contextual understanding of specific situations, and focuses on such rudimentary moral skills as kindness, sensitivity, attentiveness, tact, patience, and reliability. Earlier theories, including social contract theory, assumed that the norm of justice provided an adequate framework of universal rules for the moral dimensions of professional practice. Justice ethics reduces relations between individuals to a consideration of only those universal rights possessed by all persons, and then applies universal rules, ignoring all context.[3] In espousing a "perspective of care," Gilligan identifies a moral dimension in human relationships and the responsiveness that arises between human beings who see themselves as being unique rather than abstractly conceived rights-bearers. In Gilligan's view, moral questions cannot be comprehended solely by the justice-based demands of equality, impartiality, and universality; rather, her "perspective of care" allows partiality to emerge as a legitimate moral point of view.[4] Indeed, the ethics of care requires an accurate understanding of moral competence, including the skills and forms of human relating.

## Traditional ethical theories applied to the practice of pharmacy

In the early 1930s, C. D. Broad brought ancient and modern ethical theories into a unified classification scheme, distinguishing two basic types of ethical theory that are still serviceable today: *Consequentialism*, an ethical theory concerned only with the outcomes or consequences of actions, and *nonconsequentialism*, an ethical theory based upon the actions themselves without particular regard to their consequences.[5] To a consequentialist, an action becomes "right" or "wrong" in terms of the benefit or harm the patient—and all others concerned—might derive from a given action. Following this line of reasoning, lying to a patient would be permissible, even laudable, if it resulted in some benefit to the patient or others. This rather paternalistic approach to patient care is the major principle underlying the Hippocratic Oath and the many other codes of professional conduct that have been developed by pharmacists and physicians during the last 150 years.

The nonconsequentialist, on the other hand, looks at the action itself as either right or wrong, without regard to outcome. Following this line of reasoning, lying to a patient is wrong by definition, whether or not the lie might ultimately "benefit" all concerned parties. Pharmacists who deeply believe in nonconsequentialism are devoted to being faithful to the patient above all other considerations and are therefore disposed to tell the truth in even the most sensitive situations. These pharmacists would speak frankly, but kindly, to terminal cancer patients who are apparently unaware of the seriousness of their condition, confident that they are being faithful to them. In contrast, pharmacists who believe in consequentialism must struggle deciding whether the false serenity resulting from lying to these same patients would be more beneficial than any anguish resulting from telling the truth. To the pharmacist guided by nonconsequentialism, this dilemma is simply not an issue. Nonconsequentialism tends to be less paternalistic by allowing its proponents to focus upon a more objective goal—telling the truth becomes a "good" that outweighs the consequences associated with telling the truth or the patient's ability to handle the truth.

In applying these theories to ethical dilemmas, many philosophers appeal to widely accepted moral standards in their quest for acceptable outcomes. These standards include *beneficence*, the principle that guides the actions and behaviors of practitioners toward beneficial patient outcomes, and *nonmaleficence*, the principle that urges practitioners to avoid actions and behaviors that might bring harm to their patients. Pharmacists demonstrate beneficence whenever they provide critically needed prescription drugs to their patients in emergency situations without regard to possible legal consequences. Pharmacists who refuse to fill a prescription order because of their concern for patient safety or well-being observe the principle of nonmaleficence. Beneficence and nonmaleficence are addressed more fully in Chapter 3 in the context of the pharmacist-patient relationship.

## Newer ethical principles applied to the practice of pharmacy

Within the last two decades, the conceptual foundation for evaluating outcomes within the tenets of consequentialism has been expanded to include other ethical principles beyond beneficence and nonmaleficence. These newer principles press the practitioner-patient relationship beyond these traditional ethical guidelines to include such additional principles as *justice*, strategies or acts that ensure the fair allocation of goods and services, *autonomy*, strategies or acts that respect the self-determination of other persons, and *fidelity*, strategies or acts that stress faithfulness and promise-keeping. While the pharmacist-patient relationships associated with these newer principles are discussed in some detail in Chapter 3, it may be useful to distinguish them here.

Pharmacists driven by *justice* attempt to treat all their patients with equanimity and fairness, regardless of circumstances or the likelihood of their patients benefitting from a certain therapy or even being able to pay for it. Pharmacists who respect the *autonomy* of their patients will never attempt to interfere with their patient's right of self-determination or influence the patient's decisions by withholding or shading drug product information that might result in a patient's noncompliance or discontinuing needed therapy. Finally, pharmacists who display a strong sense of *fidelity* will always maintain their patient's diagnoses, laboratory test results, prescription records, and other clinical information in the strictest confidence. These pharmacists also display their faithfulness by embracing related virtues such as *truthfulness* as an integral part of their covenant with their patients and strive toward absolute honesty and promise-keeping.

## Character and virtue in the practice of pharmacy

A second possible conceptual basis for ethical practice in pharmacy involves studying the underlying virtues of its practitioners and the traits of character most often associated with these virtues. *Virtue* is often defined in term of traits of character that are valued as a human quality; that is, by looking at the virtues of individuals, we are able to gauge their character, and can better understand the attitudes with which they approach moral decisions. "If a virtuous person makes a mistake in judgment, thereby performing a morally wrong act, he or she would be less blameworthy than an habitual offender who performed the same act," ethicists Tom Beauchamp and James Childress declare.[6] While society can forgive a virtuous person who makes a poor ethical choice on occasion, it is much less forgiving of errors made by persons it considers nonvirtuous or patent scoundrels. Such virtues as *faithfulness, fortitude, tenderness*, and *compassion* have been associated with—and in some cases driven—the moral motivations of health-care practitioners for centuries. The traditional Confucian virtues of *humaneness, compassion*, and *filial piety*, for example, so dominate the attitudes of Chinese physicians that they often place a higher value upon being a virtuous person than producing a morally correct outcome. By the same token, Sir Thomas Percival's insistence that the early nineteenth-century English physician display *"tenderness* with *steadiness"* and *"condescension* with *authority"* reflects his contention that a physician be a gentleman first; if the physician is a gentleman, he will make good ethical decisions by virtue of simply being a gentleman.[7]

The premise that the virtuous person will make morally defensible decisions, of course, may be incorrect: a physician who purposefully avoids telling a patient he has a terminal illness out of a sense of compassion may violate that patient's right to self-determination; a pharmacist who tolerates the potential dangers associated with a drug-impaired colleague out of a sense of loyalty or faithfulness may neglect his ethical duty to keep patients from harm. This distinction has profound implications for health-care practitioners: because virtues are held by individuals, they reflect the unique beliefs of individuals. This means that practitioners can not only hold different virtues, but can assign different levels of importance to the same virtue. Pharmacists who hold justice as a primal principle guiding their practice will provide professional services without regard to external constraints placed upon those services. Such pharmacists will provide their professional services in an equitable manner without regard to the age, sex, or appearance of their patients, or even their ability to pay for their services. Other pharmacists, guided by a different primal principle, such as steadfastness, might refuse service to a certain class of clientele or refuse to fill welfare prescriptions or extend credit, but still might be widely regarded as virtuous practitioners who can always be depended upon to be helpful and supportive to their patients.

**The role of virtue in pharmacy practice.** Despite the ambiguities associated with relying upon virtue and character in ethical decision-making, American pharmacy has reflected a long tradition of virtuous, responsible behavior. In 1821, founders of the Philadelphia College of Pharmacy saw their new local association as a "timely and effectual remedy" for maintaining the "respectability" of their emerging profession and urged new members to display "correct moral deportment." In his 1857 paper, "Ethical Analysis," Edward Parrish declared that "actions in themselves right are never incompatible with each other; they have always a favorable effect upon the integrity of the individual; they improve and elevate his instincts and affections, and put him in harmony with the good and the true." Nearly a century later, the deeply probing *General Report of the Pharmaceutical Survey* (1950) concluded that "the outstanding factor determining the future of the profession of pharmacy is fundamentally moral in nature."[8]

What virtues do present-day pharmacists find to be the most important in their practice? Baldwin and Alberts suggest that honesty, dedication, carefulness, and dependability must command consideration.[9] The American Association of Colleges of Nursing provides an extensive list of essential values and attitudes including commitment, generosity, tolerance, empathy, integrity, kindness, and rationality (see Table 2.1). Moreover, as the process of professionalization within the practice of pharmacy and the goals of modern health care have become more fully realized, society appears to have identified a number of specific virtues within contemporary pharmacy practice. For example, the Gallup Poll tells us that over two-thirds of Americans rank nurses and pharmacists as the most respected of all professionals on the basis of honesty and ethical standards.[10] While the underlying reasons for these high

Table 2.1. Values and Behaviors for Professional Pharmacists[*]

| Values | Attitudes | Professional Behavior |
| --- | --- | --- |
| Altruism (concern for the welfare of others) | Commitment Compassion Generosity | Gives full attention to patients Assists other health-care personnel Sensitive to social issues |
| Equality (having the same rights, privileges, or status) | Fairness Self-esteem Tolerance | Provides services based on needs Relates to others without discriminating Provides leadership in improving access to health care |
| Esthetics (qualities of objects, events, and persons that provide satisfaction) | Appreciation Creativity Sensitivity | Creates supportive patient-care environments |
| Freedom (capacity to exercise choice) | Openness Self-direction Self-discipline | Respects each individual's autonomy |
| Human Dignity (inherent worth and uniqueness of an individual) | Empathy Kindness Trust | Respects the right of privacy Maintains confidentiality |
| Justice (upholding moral and legal principles) | Integrity Morality | Acts as a health-care advocate Allocates resources fairly Reports incompetent, unethical, and illegal practices |
| Truth (faithfulness to fact or reality) | Accountability Honesty Rationality | Documents actions accurately Protects the public from misinformation about pharmacy |

[*]Adopted from *Essentials of College and University Education for Professional Nursing: Final Report* (Washington, D.C.: American Association of Colleges of Nursing, 1986), pp. 6-7.

ratings remain somewhat of a mystery, Americans evidently feel very comfortable entrusting a portion of their health-care needs to their pharmacists.

**Commonly held virtues among pharmacists.** While pharmacists have displayed a wide range of virtues in their practice, most of these virtues can be discussed under three broad categories: *fair dealing and equity, patient-centered services,* and *faithfulness.* It is significant that all three of these virtues have been incorporated in nearly every version of the Code of Ethics of the American Pharmaceutical Association.

*Fair dealing and equity.* Pharmacists have traditionally taken great pride in being fair and equitable in both their professional and their business dealings with patients, other pharmacists, and physicians. The earliest Code of Ethics of the American Pharmaceutical Association (1852) enjoined pharmacists to "discountenance quackery" in their dealings with customers and avoid "dishonorable competition" in their relationships with each other. Business intrigues with physicians were held not only as "unprofessional and highly reprehensible" and "unjust to the public," but "hurtful to the independence and self-respect" of both parties.[11] It seems clear that the framers of this Code wished to see pharmacists held to a higher standard of personal behavior than other mid-nineteenth-century American shopkeepers. Indeed, a preoccupation with fair business dealings seems to be a hallmark of most early codes of pharmacy ethics. Later versions of the Code (1922, 1952) continued to stress adherence to fair business practices, banning such seemingly unsavory practices as filling coded prescriptions, imitating labels of competitors, filling orders intended for competitors, or soliciting professional practice through advertising. The 1981 version of the Code enjoined pharmacists to "seek at all times only fair and reasonable remuneration for professional services" and never engage in financial practices that may cause "financial or other exploitation in connection with the rendering of professional services." In contrast, the 1994 Code of Ethics for Pharmacists simply states that "a pharmacist acts with honesty and integrity in professional relationships."[12]

*Patient-centered services.* The 1922 Code of Ethics of the Association defined the pharmacist's relationship to the public in terms of "safeguarding the handling, sale, compounding, and dispensing of medicinal substances." The pharmacist was exhorted to "hold the health and safety of his patrons to be of first consideration" and "regulate his public and private conduct and deeds so as to entitle him to the respect and confidence of the community in which he practices." As the focus of pharmacy practice began to shift from product-centered to patient-centered values, the 1981 Code urged the pharmacist to "render to each patient the full measure of professional ability as an essential health practitioner." The 1994 Code of Ethics for Pharmacists states that "a pharmacist promotes the good of every patient," a broader standard that places "concern for the well-being of the patient at the center of professional practice."[13] Today, the tensions that emerge from attempting to balance the human and patient-centered values of a health profession with the very real and practical demands of the business world test the value system of even the most dedicated pharmacist.

*Faithfulness.* The 1922 Code of Ethics calls upon the pharmacist to "enlist and merit the confidence of his patrons," adding that once this confidence is established, it should be "jealously guarded and never abused by extortion or misrepresentation in any other manner." The Code further considered the knowledge and confidences associated with the ailments of a pharmacist's patients as "entrusted to his honor," exhorting the pharmacist to "never divulge such facts unless compelled to do so by law." By 1969, the Code carried this appeal to faithfulness beyond mere compliance with the law noting that the pharmacist "should not disclose such information to anyone without proper patient authorization." In studied contrast, the 1994 Code of Ethics for Pharmacists recognizes the pharmacist-patient relationship as a "covenant," and places further emphasis on faithfulness by emphasizing that "a pharmacist focuses on serving the patient in a private and confidential manner."[14]

## Rights and duties in the practice of pharmacy

The third and most emotionally charged conceptual basis for ethical pharmacy practice lies in the realm of human rights and professional duties and the inherent tension that can exist between these concepts. The importance of human rights as reflected in the tenets of liberal individualism has emerged as a driving force in American society. During the last two decades, societal claims to the right to know, the right to die, the right to privacy, and the right to health care has transformed nearly every aspect of personal and professional life. "Health care can no longer be a private matter to be purchased as any other market commodity," bioethicist George H. Kieffer declares. "Rather, health care must be considered a necessary *social* resource like education or police protection."[15] In response to this societal mandate, nearly every institution and professional association within the health-care field has embraced the notion of "patient rights" to some extent. The American Hospital Association's vaunted "Patient's Bill of Rights" (1992), for example, attempts to articulate specific rights that hospitalized patients might claim, suggesting that the physician is required, by claim of right, to involve his patients in nearly every aspect of the decision-making process associated with their therapy. This new claim—and the underlying respect it may command as either a "natural" or "bestowed" right—moves the physician-patient relationship far beyond the typical bounds of the paternalistic Hippocratic Oath. In 1992, the National Association of Boards of Pharmacy (NABP) encouraged the promulgation of a "Pharmacy Patient's Bill of Rights," in acknowledgment of an "increasingly informed and cost-conscious public," making specific reference to the "proliferation and complexity of drug therapy." The document was developed to provide pharmacists with "a common reference to describe their covenental relationship with the public."[16]

**Understanding rights.** *Rights* may be defined as justified claims that individuals or groups can make on others or upon society. Rights emanate from two distinct sources: *natural rights*—such as the right to life, the right to freedom, and the right to die—which are inherent to the human condition, and *bestowed rights*—such as the right to a living wage, the right to privacy, and the right to health care—which must be granted by others—a government, institution, or individuals. Rights may be further divided into *legal rights*—rights established through regulations, legislation, or court decisions and enforced by such sanctions as fines or imprisonment—and *moral rights*—rights established through commonly held religious tenets or cultural mores.

Rights not only form a significantly symbolic underpinning to our society, but also exert a powerful force in the development of our system of health care. Since the turn of the present century, an increasing number of Americans have claimed the "right" to a wide gamut of governmentally assured health-care services, including the "right" to receive exotic and expensive technological procedures, the "right" to choose their own health-care providers, and the "right" to obtain prescription drugs through such programs as Medicare and Medicaid. Philosopher Norman Daniels notes that these claims imply a variety of related societal duties, such as the duty to allocate an adequate share of total resources to health-related needs and the duty to provide a just allocation of different types of health services while providing each individual a fair share of such services.[17] To the extent that these "rights" have been fulfilled and promulgated into law as bestowed rights, they have had a profound impact upon the practice of medicine and pharmacy.

**Understanding duties.** Every right carries with it an obligation on someone else to behave in a certain manner. This obligation to perform some prescribed conduct is referred to as a *duty*. The natural right of freedom, for example, carries with it a corresponding duty to not abridge that freedom. The bestowed right of health-care assistance to the indigent through Medicaid implies an obligation on all health-care practitioners to provide that assistance in an equitable manner. Specific examples of duties related to the practice of pharmacy include the duty to be faithful to one's patients, the duty to tell them the truth, and the duty to treat their medication records in a confidential manner.

Some moral philosophers argue that rights follow duty; that is, once a duty is fully accepted it establishes a right. Ethicists refer to the rather confusing relationship between rights and duties as the *correlativity of rights*. To complicate matters further, the term "duty" is often used imprecisely to refer to acts driven by conscience, religious beliefs, or social mores.[18] In addition, individuals may face situations that present conflicting duties: For example, pharmacists who feel a duty to warn patients about the possible complications of specific drug therapy may also feel an equally strong obligation to withhold such information because it might undermine the physician-patient relationship or otherwise interfere with the intended therapeutic outcomes. Pharmacists faced with such dilemmas must resolve the apparent conflict among these duties by deciding which of these competing duties claims a higher priority within the framework of their personal value system.

## Professional Codes as a Framework for Decision-Making

Self-regulation and self-discipline are generally regarded by society as essential requisites for a profession, particularly those professions that are associated with maintaining and extending the health and well-being of individuals within the society. As we have noted in Chapter 1, professionals are given certain legal privileges by society, including a quasi-monopoly to practice within a certain professional arena. In return for these privileges, professionals accept the responsibility to maintain a standard of conduct beyond either an unthinking conformity to the law or the perfunctory performance of a technical skill. This common concern for collective self-discipline encompasses the very essence of a *professional ethic*; indeed, a professional ethic is one of several generally accepted criteria that serve to distinguish a profession from other occupations.

This ethic is generally promulgated by professional associations in the form of a *code of ethics*, a detailed, explicit, operational blueprint of norms of professional conduct, a public recital of desirable and undesirable actions having an impact upon the character of a profession and its functional reliability. Medieval guilds and, later, professional associations wrote restrictive codes of conduct that reflected their collective values and aspirations to self-determination rather than relying upon the more stringent and less desirable controls imposed by legislation and social sanctions. In the United States, both the 1848 code of ethics of the Philadelphia College of Pharmacy, which attempted to advance "professional conduct and probity" to correspond to the "standard of scientific attainments" it felt it had achieved, and the 1852 code of the American Pharmaceutical Association (APhA), modeled after the Philadelphia example, which asked those who honored it to "protect themselves and the public from the ill effect of an undue competition, and the temptation to gain at the expense of quality," established guidelines for professional practice far beyond the realities of everyday practice.[19] In so doing, the associations created a pattern of lofty professional aspirations that persists to this day. Nevertheless, professional codes of ethics have stood the test of time and have generally not only exerted a positive, cohesive force upon individual members of a profession, but also served as a publicly proclaimed benchmark for a standard of professional conduct above and beyond minimal legal and social expectations.

## Difficulties associated with traditional codes

As products of professional associations, codes of ethics reflect the consensus of a wide range of individual practitioners' opinions on an equally wide range of real or potential practice dilemmas at a particular point in time. These consensus statements also mirror changes in practice standards rather than standing alone as an unswerving, underlying moral philosophy. For example, the pressures exerted upon pharmacists in the years following the enactment of federal narcotic legislation and national prohibition prompted a detailed reference to the "dispensing and sale of narcotic drugs and alcoholic liquors" in the 1922 Code of the APhA. Similarly, the 1952 revision of the APhA Code reflected the emergence of brand-name pharmaceutical products and subsequent state-based antisubstitution laws, as it urged pharmacists to recognize the "significance and legal aspects of brand names and trade-marked products," but made no mention of the then moot "alcoholic liquor" issue.

The thought that professional codes are dictated by ever-changing problems and circumstances, promulgated by professional groups who may be merely promoting their own self-interest is deeply disturbing. "If professional ethics mean nothing more than those behaviors required by the professional group," ethicist Robert M. Veatch rumbles, "then it is logically impossible to say that one's professional group has taken a morally incorrect stand."[20] While the 1994 Code of Ethics for Pharmacists attempts to overcome these objections by focusing upon patient care, professional codes of ethics have a number of other difficulties as well, which we will explore below.

**Codes are not all-encompassing.** By their very nature, most professional codes of ethics are self-limited and restricted in scope. Brief codes of ethics are too abstract or idealized to be useful and may avoid dealing with sensitive areas. Such codes are designed primarily for their public relations value and are usually described as being "suitable for framing and display in your place of practice." The ideal code of ethics usually consists of a concise, generalized code supplemented by a manual of interpretations or case histories. Medicine, nursing, and law now use this latter approach, which is also intended to be developed for the 1994 Code of Ethics for Pharmacists as this Code becomes fully implemented.

Appeal to a professional code of ethics for assistance in decision-making during a difficult ethical dilemma may produce results that are less than useful. Often, the elements of the code are so universal in scope that they are of little practical value as an action guide for resolving difficult dilemmas in practice. For example, pharmacy codes of ethics do not include any specific rules to help the pharmacist deal with patients who request additional medication before their usual refill interval, or how to handle medical emergencies typified by the frantic patient staggering to the prescription area, clutching his arm, and pleading, "Please, give me some nitroglycerin for my angina!" These specific examples are encompassed by such generalized statements in the 1981 APhA Code of Ethics as "the pharmacist should hold the health and safety of patients to be of first consideration," and can lead to a wide range of different individual interpretations, each of which may be internally logical and consistent. Other practitioners, noting a subsequent statement that "the pharmacist has the duty to observe the law" can choose a very narrow, linear, or legalistic interpretation of the Code and refuse to provide such emergency services.

**Codes may be ambiguous.** Codes of professional ethics also tend to be vague and not easily applied to practice situations. Often, in attempting to encompass a wide range of professional behavior within the confines of a series of generalized, inspirational statements, the framers of codes of ethics invariably produce irritatingly ambiguous statements that are of little practical value to practitioners seeking guidance in solving specific ethical problems in practice. Pharmacists seeking assistance in solving difficult questions of information disclosure are often disappointed in their attempts to use codes of professional ethics for guidance. The 1981 APhA Code of Ethics, for example, expects the pharmacist to "respect the confidential and personal nature of professional records," but offers an exception "where the best interest of the patient requires," thus allowing pharmacists to determine when the "best interest of the patient" requires a breach of confidentiality.

**Codes are difficult to enforce.** When the American Pharmaceutical Association was formed in 1852, members were accepted on the basis of subscribing to its new Code of Ethics, but American pharmacy was not ready to adhere to such rigid standards. APhA Secretary Edward Parrish concluded that these ethical rules had to be a goal, but not a condition for membership. The obligation to subscribe to the APhA Code as a prerequisite of membership was dropped in 1855 and the Code itself disappeared from the literature for over a half a century, even though members were expelled from time to time for "violation of APhA's sense of moral rectitude and the general purposes of its organization."[21] In 1922, the APhA adopted a new and comprehensive Code of Ethics based upon the fundamental relationships of the pharmacist with the public, the physician, and fellow practitioners. This version of the Code and its 1952 revision were presumably to be enforced by peer pressure and individual practitioners' consciences, for no mechanism existed within the Association for securing adherence to its principles. In

1966, the Association established a Judicial Board empowered to "discipline members and render advisory opinions and interpretive statements, reprimanding, suspending or expelling a member in any category . . . for unprofessional conduct."[22] Unfortunately, the Board did not survive the first serious challenge to its new authority. In 1970, the Board received a complaint regarding advertising of prescription services by two pharmacy chains in Michigan, citing a provision in the Code requiring that pharmacists "not solicit professional practice by means of advertising." In its attempt to enforce this ban against advertising, the Board became embroiled in a lawsuit that resulted in a temporary injunction prohibiting it from taking further action against the chains, effectively nullifying the Board's enforcement power. Moreover, the publicity surrounding the lawsuit drew the attention of federal agencies to the dispute, causing the Association to revise this section of the Code to be more circumspect of the federal antitrust laws.[23]

State boards of pharmacy in Pennsylvania, New Jersey, and elsewhere have also attempted to enforce professional standards by incorporating elements of their state association's code of ethics into their statutes or regulations. Other state pharmacy practice acts set forth "unprofessional conduct" as a basis for suspension or revocation of a pharmacist's license. While legal enforcement of ethical standards may be a tempting solution to a knotty professional problem, these statutes and regulations are often vaguely worded and may grant the board of pharmacy an overly broad area of discretion. For these reasons, attempts to enforce ethical standards through legal mechanisms have not withstood judicial scrutiny.[24]

**Codes usually lack patient input.** Framers of early codes of pharmacy ethics also presumed that their codes reflected their patients' best interests; as such, they developed language describing pharmacists' behavior toward their patients and the benefits the patients would derive from that behavior, all without consulting the patient. The presumption that professional associations can speak authoritatively to patients' needs without consulting the patients themselves not only smacks of paternalism, but jeopardizes the credibility of the codes themselves. The wave of consumerism in the 1970s brought with it not only an increased public interest in prescription pricing policies and access to drug information, but also an increased interest in professional accountability, reflected by the appointment of lay members to state boards of pharmacy, a province traditionally restricted to practitioners.[25] Unfortunately, this increased interest in professional accountability did not extend into the realm of professional ethics, for codes of ethics continue to be drafted by well-meaning committees of professional associations without the benefit of meaningful input from representatives of the public. It is difficult, for example, to conceive of a lay member approving "ethical" rules prohibiting advertising or discounting of prescription prices as anything more than self-serving statements designed to limit competition or guarantee pharmacists' incomes. Nevertheless, despite the generally positive and open atmosphere engendered in pharmacy by the consumerism movement, lay participation in drafting codes of professional conduct remains an elusive goal in pharmacy and all other health-care professions as well.

## A Framework for Ethical Decision-Making in Pharmacy Practice

Given some understanding of the four major systems that form the foundation for ethical decision-making, we can turn our attention to the process of making these decisions in our professional practice. In *Human Values in Health Care: The Practice of Ethics*, philosopher Richard A. Wright developed a four-step framework for assessing ethical situations. More recently, pharmacy professor Jack Justice introduced a ten-step model for resolving ethical dilemmas in pharmacy practice based upon objectivity and critical thinking.[26] Both models view ethical decision-making as a generalizable problem-solving process that can be easily learned. We propose a more modest but equally serviceable four-step problem-solving process: *identify the problem, consider alternative courses of action, select one alternative,* and *consider objections* to the alternative selected. This process not only encourages pharmacists to make professional decisions based on reflection and reason, but also ensures that the resulting choice is validated in ethical terms.

### Step one: Problem identification

The first step in the problem-solving process—problem identification—may appear deceptively simple. Nevertheless, the clear identification of an ethical problem sets the stage for systematic problem analysis. It goes without saying that the problem you identify should have an ethical basis and not be rooted in legal issues or professional courtesies. George H. Kieffer stresses that problem identification must be "as clear as possible in order to reduce uncertainty and ambiguity."[27] A mental checklist for problem identification includes four distinct steps: *identify technical facts*, *identify moral parameters*, *identify legal constraints*, and *identify relevant human values*.

**Identify technical facts.** The first step in problem identification is the straightforward collection of data: who are the people involved in the dilemma, both directly and indirectly? The pharmacist, patient, and physician are surely involved in most cases, but to what extent will your decisions affect your employer, your patient's family, or other physicians? To what extent, for example, do your personal moral standards color your ethical decisions? Every ethical dilemma consists of a myriad of smaller choices, each of which has a value associated with it. Some of these value judgments may not be germane to the case in point; nevertheless, each of these choices must be assessed within the context of the overall ethical dilemma and not considered as isolated decision points. Thus, your development of a truly useful data base for ethical decision-making depends upon your assessment of the total fact situation.

**Identify moral parameters.** Once you have identified and assessed all of the facts associated with a given ethical problem, you can proceed to identify and distinguish the moral dilemmas and ethical issues that are associated with the problem. To what extent, for example, does a competitive pricing policy affect all segments of your clientele? Filling prescriptions for oral contraceptives below cost may be dismissed as an unsavory business practice frowned upon in many codes of ethics, but hardly merits moral reasoning. Making up for this loss by increasing your professional fee on maintenance medication, however, involves the issue of justice, particularly if this policy adversely affects one specific group of your patients. Finally, be aware that your personal bias can color your assessment of moral issues. Thus, pharmacists who inveigh long and loud against all social welfare programs may be less than candid in assessing the issues of fairness or justice that naturally arise from such programs.

**Identify legal constraints.** The next step in the problem identification process involves identifying to what extent legal constraints might affect your assessment of the problem. In some states, for example, the confidentiality of patient prescription records is assured by statute. In this instance, pharmacists faced with the decision of whether or not to discuss a patient's medical records with a third party need merely observe the law and not consider the moral or ethical parameters associated with patient confidentiality. In the past, many pharmacists sought to solve many of their professional or ethical problems through such legislation. As noted in Chapter 3, the appeal to the legislative process to resolve professional dilemmas may be taken as one sign of the incomplete professionalization of an occupation. Finally, whereas some ethical problems may be resolved by illegal acts—supplying an unauthorized nitroglycerin tablet to the proverbial angina patient—ethical pharmacists would ordinarily appeal to the law first for guidance in making their professional decisions.

**Identify relevant human values.** The final—and in many cases the most important—step in problem identification involves developing a detailed account of the human values associated with each ethical dilemma identified. Human values not only help pharmacists frame their ethical problems, but may also suggest alternatives for resolution of the problem. In fact, our values actually determine whether or not we even see an ethical problem as a problem. For example, pharmacists confronted with an angry demand from a father for confidential information about his adolescent daughter's medications need to consider not only their personal set of values and the values incorporated in a code of ethics, but also the values exhibited by the person making the demand. In this case, the father may be strongly motivated by other competing values such as his loyalty to his daughter or his duty to protect her from possible harm. Pharmacists who can identify and understand the wide gamut of human values present in a given professional dilemma are better prepared to make judgments that provide the foundation for defensible ethical decision-making.

## Step two: Develop alternative courses of action

The second step in the problem-solving process—developing alternative courses of action—is inherently difficult for students and practitioners alike. In many cases, one and only one alternative leaps to the mind, while other alternatives are discarded as not meriting serious consideration. In contrast, it should be possible to establish an exhaustive list of alternative actions for each ethical dilemma that arises. The purpose of listing alternative actions is not merely an academic exercise, but rather a plea for thoroughness in deciding which of several equally satisfying actions should be taken. Informed ethical decision-making promotes informed choices rather than instinctive reactions, resulting in decisions based on reason, rather than urgency.

**Identify relevant ethical principles for each alternative.** Just as it is important to identify all the technical facts associated with an ethical dilemma, it is equally important to identify all the relevant ethical principles associated with each alternative. These mutually exclusive alternatives often reveal competing ethical principles, each of which may suggest diverse solutions to the problem. In the situation outlined above, the pharmacist confronted by an angry father faces a number of clear choices: If he chooses to supply the information, he shows a lack of respect for the autonomy of the daughter; if he evades the request by referring the father to his daughter's physician, he ignores the values of the father; if he lies by telling the father he does not have the information, he may sacrifice his own personal values with regard to truth-telling.

**Recognize ethical assumptions for each alternative.** Each alternative action may have a number of "ethical assumptions" associated with it. By ethical assumptions we refer to the supposition that one or more moral principles are inherent to a particular case. In the above example, the pharmacist who chooses to tell the truth operates on the ethical assumption that all pharmacists are honest and trustworthy and would therefore never lie to their patients. The Gallup Poll paints an attractive picture of the "trusted pharmacist," suggesting that honesty is a widely-held standard of professional conduct among pharmacists, lending great credibility to such an assumption. Unfortunately, we all know pharmacists who may not merit our complete trust, undercutting the assumption that *all* pharmacists are trustworthy. As we consider the wide range of action alternatives open to us, we should also consider the soundness of the ethical assumptions upon which these actions are based.

**Determine additional emerging ethical problems.** As we consider and analyze each action alternative, we also expand the field of ethical inquiry. For example, the pharmacist who decides to provide confidential information to the angry father faces an additional ethical dilemma: should he inform the daughter of his action or remain silent, hoping to avoid another unpleasant confrontation with the daughter? Other ethical issues may emerge as an indirect result of this exhaustive ethical decision-making process: Consider the feelings of the daughter's physician who might resent any intrusion into the physician-patient relationship or the feelings of the pharmacist's employer who might be concerned about the loss of a long-time customer. The possibility of linkages between action alternatives and other unanticipated ethical problems underscores the importance of viewing each ethical dilemma in the broadest possible context.

## Step three: Select one alternative course of action

The third and most satisfying step in the problem-solving process involves selecting the one action alternative that best fits your personal and professional value system. Although selecting one of several equally attractive competing alternatives may be troubling, the sense of fulfillment and professional well-being associated with resolving a complicated ethical problem provides its own reward. You should, however, be able to justify your selection and defend it upon ethical grounds.

**Justify the selection of your alternative.** Sound ethical decisions are grounded in equally sound moral justifications, such as principles, virtues, rights, or theories. In selecting your action alternative, it is imperative that you be able to identify the specific foundation upon which you made your selection and the process of reasoning which led you to your conclusion. Ask yourself the question, "Why did I make this particular selection?" This internal dialogue lies at the heart of the decision-making process, removing the possibility that you were operating upon mere whim. Moreover, you should be able to explain why the other possibilities you identified were discarded and why. Recall that more than one action may be acceptable in a given situation.

**Defend your selection upon ethical grounds.** It is especially important that you are able to provide a moral foundation for selecting the action alternative that will ultimately guide your ethical decision-making. Sometimes your selection may be founded upon several competing moral principles, each of which carries its own unique string of consequences. For example, a pharmacist may have to choose between honoring fidelity to a patient and loyalty to a physician, two principles solidly grounded in moral tradition. Whenever you are faced with deciding between competing moral principles or values, you should be able to explain why you chose one alternative over another.

## Step four: Consider objections to alternative selected

The fourth and final step in the problem-solving process involves anticipating any objections that might arise as the result of your ethical decision. Ethical dilemmas are usually complex situations involving several individuals, each with their own unique value system. Such complexity invariably breeds a wide diversity of opinion; as a result, any given action alternative will have its critics. On the other hand, the obvious "ethical outrage" generates little, if any, controversy. For example, a pharmacist who defends fraudulent welfare billing on the basis of sluggish claims processing or a surgeon who initiates adventuresome procedures unauthorized by the patient is usually condemned by all parties involved.[28] Fortunately, we rarely encounter an ethical outrage in practice; most of the ethical dilemmas we face can generate a wide range of objections. These objections usually arise from three sources: factual errors, faulty reasoning, and conflicting values.

**Objections arising from factual errors.** Pharmacists are taught to pay close attention to details and are usually fact-oriented by nature; as a result, they can usually easily identify the relevant facts in an ethical dilemma. With practice, both pharmacists and students should be able to minimize or eliminate factual errors in any ethical analysis. Most factual errors can be avoided by first carefully assessing the situation and then rigorously applying the problem-solving skills outlined above. Practice with the decision-making process using ethical dilemmas as the focus will also provide some insulation against making factual errors.

**Objections arising from faulty reasoning.** Eliminating factual errors in your ethical analysis is an important first step; eliminating faulty reasoning in your analysis is somewhat more challenging. You must be able to justify the action alternative you have chosen on the criteria of both *relevancy* and *sufficiency*. That is, the reasons you choose to justify your action alternative must not only be relevant to the situation at hand, but the reasons behind your choice must be sufficiently convincing. For example, if you decide to tell the truth in a given situation, you must also be able to state the reasons why you chose to tell the truth. To justify your choice with personal standards—"My mother always told me to tell the truth"—may be relevant, but may not be sufficient. Community standards, religious beliefs, and statements from a code of ethics may be sufficient to bolster your choice.

Objections arising from conflicting values. As noted in Chapter 1, there are very few, if any, value-free decisions in contemporary pharmacy practice. As a result, we might expect other practitioners to challenge our decisions with equally valid, carefully reasoned, ethical choices of their own, each based upon their individual value system. Ethical dilemmas related to allocation of scarce or costly medical resources are particularly vulnerable to conflicting value systems. For example, should all patients suffering cardiac occlusion receive the latest thrombolytic drug regardless of its cost, or should this drug be reserved only for those patients who are able to pay for this new genetically engineered wonder? If our value system placed a high priority upon the health and well-being of individual patients, we would choose wide access; if our value system placed a high priority upon actions that benefit the entire community rather than the individual, we might very well decide to restrict access.

## Applying the Ethical Decision-Making Framework

Given some knowledge of four primary theoretical foundations that can assist the ethical decision-making process—ethical theories and principles, character and virtue, rights and duties, and professional codes—and a general understanding of a process model for reaching these decisions, we may now turn our attention to ethical decision-making in pharmacy practice. Just as pharmacy practice takes place in a real-world setting, our ethical decision-making is affected by such external influences as professional authority, technical competence, rules, professional values, and economic forces. Thus, ethical decision-making involves more than applying rather sterile theoretical principles to a generalized problem-solving model. It must be done in the context of real-life situations facing the pharmacist. For this reason, the following cases will be discussed in the broad context of contemporary pharmacy practice. Case 2.1 illustrates how ethical decisions can be influenced by professional authority; it also provides a fully developed example of how one might use the ethical analysis model outlined above.

### Decisions influenced by professional authority

As integral members of the health-care team, pharmacists continually evaluate the prescribing practices of physicians and other prescribers to ensure optimal therapeutic outcomes for their patients. New drug entities, new therapeutic indications, and other changes in recommended prescribing regimens offer excellent opportunities for pharmacists to serve as therapeutic advisors to the physician-prescriber. Unfortunately, the role of therapeutic advisor can also lead to dissonance and conflict when pharmacists and physicians disagree over the best way to treat a particular patient. The following case illustrates one such conflict.

### Case 2.1: Conflicts in Therapy

*"Are you trying to tell me how to practice medicine?"*

Dan Smith, a newly licensed pharmacist, was settling into the rigors of professional pharmacy practice in a community medical center when he encountered a new and perplexing challenge. Dr. Tom Bond, a popular area physician and board-certified pathologist on the staff of the local community hospital, began assisting his physician-wife on a part-time basis in her practice of family medicine. His charming and beguiling manners quickly endeared him to his patients and led to an ever-increasing caseload. Unfortunately, Dr. Bond developed eccentric and sometimes dangerous medication plans: He prescribed antibiotics for unusual indications, often in subtherapeutic doses; he prescribed adult-strength cough syrups for children using adult dosage schedules; he also prescribed potent analgesics to nearly all his patients. This continuing stream of apparent "therapeutic misadventures" troubled Dan, but when he enquired about it, his pharmacist-supervisor advised him simply to comply with the orders, since Dr. Bond was ultimately responsible. Dan continued to be bothered by these peculiar orders, and decided to speak to Dr. Bond personally, hoping to either better understand his unusual treatment plans or to assist him in prescribing what Dan believed would be more appropriate drugs. After many attempts, Dan finally contacted Dr. Bond at his office and explained the nature of the call. After a few minutes of strained but polite give-and-take, Dr. Bond exploded, "Are you trying to tell me how to practice medicine?" and hung up the phone. Dan was convinced Dr. Bond would never change the way he prescribed medications, and was faced with his own personal decision about what to do next.

**Step one: Problem identification.** Dan is confronted with an ethical dilemma often encountered in pharmacy practice. What is the ethical nature of the problem that Dan is facing? What personal values might Dan hold that are relevant to the dilemma? One approach which can be used to answer these questions is to reflect upon the matter through Dan's eyes and follow his line of reasoning. At this point, for example, Dan might be thinking:

I can't allow this kind of practice to continue. If these patients knew what I know about the crazy way this doctor is prescribing, they would panic. My duty is to protect the patient from harm, or at least to make sure they understand what the drugs are going to do for them. I believe patients have a right to know the truth about the kinds of medications their doctor prescribes for them, especially if there are risks of untoward actions. If I am loyal to the patient, does that mean that I must be disloyal to the doctor? I need to talk with Dr. Bond again, but what happens if he refuses to talk to me and continues prescribing in the same manner? Can I refuse to fill his prescriptions? And if I refuse to fill his prescriptions, what should I tell his patients? Should I turn him into the medical board? And why doesn't my supervisor help me with this problem?

*Identify technical facts.* In this case, the technical facts are straightforward: Dan has witnessed this situation develop over some time; it is not an isolated instance. The situation is also apparently sanctioned by his pharmacist-supervisor, who has told Dan to "simply comply with the orders," since Dr. Bond was "ultimately responsible." From his prescription records, Dan can tell that Dr. Bond's patients appear to be loyal to him and trust themselves to his care. For Dan to suddenly refuse to fill a prescription order without an explanation would undermine the delicate trusting relationship between Dr. Bond and his patients. Finally, Dan is now quite aware of Dr. Bond's insistence that Dan not only fill his prescription orders as written, but has suggested in no uncertain terms that Dan will not be included in his therapeutic decision-making.

*Identify legal constraints.* Unfortunately, Dan's problem is neither unique nor farfetched. All pharmacists have had occasion to question whether an otherwise legally-written prescription order is therapeutically appropriate or even dangerous to the well-being of a particular patient. In this case, Dan is dealing with an extreme version of this dilemma: Although Dan tactfully attempted to present his concerns, Dr. Bond not only refused to change his prescription orders, but refused to include Dan in any form of therapeutic decision-making for his patients. The prescription was legal and appropriate therapy, Dr. Bond appeared to be saying, Dan should fill it without asking any annoying questions.

*Identify moral parameters.* Dan is responding to a value system that includes several conflicting moral issues. On one level, he is motivated by a strongly held belief in beneficence and tries to avoid bringing harm to the patients under his care. On another level, he realizes the importance of the physician-patient relationship and appears equally determined to respect this relationship. Finally, motivated by an equally strong belief in telling the truth, Dan feels compelled to try to explain to his patients the exact nature of the medications Dr. Bond has prescribed and their intended therapeutic effects. These three moral issues also tend to form the basis for describing several related human values held by Dan.

*Identify relevant human values.* Dan also appears to exhibit a value system that includes several conflicting values. While Dan certainly is committed to the ideal of beneficence, he finds that this ideal is compromised by his professional "duty" to fill Dr. Bond's prescriptions, reflecting the functional loyalty of any pharmacist to any physician. He also wishes to cause no harm to his patients—an appeal to beneficence—and realizes that it is only a matter of time before some serious injury will occur if he continues to be "loyal" to Dr. Bond. Moreover, he wishes to be honest with his patients and feels he has a duty to inform them of his concerns. Finally, Dan apparently feels both loyalty and respect for his pharmacist-supervisor and does not wish to challenge him on this sensitive issue.

**Step two: Develop alternative courses of action.** Dan has several alternative courses of action open to him: He can continue to fill Dr. Bond's unusual prescriptions, documenting his attempts to rectify the situation; he can refer Dr. Bond's patients to his pharmacist-supervisor, avoiding further personal confrontation with the problem; Dan can refuse to fill the prescriptions, telling Dr. Bond, his patients, and his supervisor exactly why he has chosen this course of action; finally, Dan can continue to fill the prescriptions without comment, disguising his reason for being concerned, and continue to seek out Dr. Bond, hoping to resolve the difficulty through an amicable compromise. You may wish to consider other alternatives beyond the realm of moral reasoning: Dan could contact the Medical Board about Dr. Bond's inappropriate prescribing habits; Dan could denounce Dr. Bond to his patients as a dangerous quack; as a last resort, Dan could resign his position as pharmacist.

**Step three: Select one alternative course of action.** It seems clear that Dan has a complex and strongly held value system that would prevent him from either taking no action, deferring the decision to his supervisor, or undermining Dr. Bond's physician-patient relationships by unsolicited truth-telling or denunciation. Moreover, at his current level of moral awareness, Dan cannot continue to fill Dr. Bond's prescriptions and merely document his unwilling compliance. Dan also realizes that Dr. Bond's wife may be able to provide care for her husband's patients if he loses his prescribing privileges, but he has serious doubts of this occurring. Finally, it would not be characteristic of Dan to refuse to fill the troublesome prescriptions and inform all parties of his concerns, despite his strong belief in beneficence and truth-telling because of the potential greater harm which could result from patients being deprived of legitimate—albeit somewhat questionable—therapy. The final action alternative—working within the system to improve Dr. Bond's prescribing habits while maintaining his patients' well-being—seems to most closely mirror Dan's value system. Moreover, this alternative provides the greatest benefit to Dan's patients by maintaining their therapy while respecting both physician-patient and pharmacist-patient relationships.

**Step four: Consider objections to alternative selected.** Dan realizes the possibility of harm to Dr. Bond's patients because of what he considers to be inappropriate therapy, but he can find no real evidence of such harm. Furthermore, Dan realizes the significance of supporting Dr. Bond's relationships with his patients; to confront Dr. Bond with a rigid attitude would cause them anxiety and a discontinuity in their care, causing needless discomfort and harm. Most troubling is Dan's decision to not inform Dr. Bond's patients of his concerns and acting solely on his own initiative. Dr. Bond's patients may have a voice to offer, and Dan's decision to resolve the dilemma without their consent ignores their right to know the potential harm from Dr. Bond's irrational prescribing. Nevertheless, Dan's decision to exclude Dr. Bond's patients from these discussions does not supersede the benefits to be gained by Dan's continued support of the physician-patient relationships.

## Decisions influenced by technical competence

Pharmacists are often sought out by the public for their expertise in both prescription and nonprescription medication. When patients ask a pharmacist for a frank opinion about a certain over-the-counter drug in which the pharmacist has full confidence, few ethical conflicts arise. Similarly, most pharmacists feel no conflict in reinforcing a physician's drug regimen to a questioning or apprehensive patient. What happens, however, when a patient asks the pharmacist's opinion about a prescribed drug the pharmacist believes is too expensive, ineffective, or otherwise inappropriate? Can pharmacists simply provide noncommittal assurance, content in the fact that they are merely filling a prescription order for which they take no real responsibility? Can a pharmacist ever justify lying to a patient? Case 2.2 examines such an issue.

### Case 2.2: Conflicts in Drug Selection

*"Is this product as good as the brand-name version?"*

Ada Pharmacy is a typical, independent pharmacy located in a small college town in northwestern Ohio. Its pharmacists pride themselves with their commitment to loyal service to their patients and are especially active in patient education. As the only pharmacy within a 25-mile radius, it serves a large population. Its pharmacists are generally viewed by its patrons to be the most reliable source of information on both prescription and nonprescription medications. Recently, Henry Lehr, the pharmacist-owner of Ada Pharmacy, has requested that all his pharmacists dispense Template Pharmaceutical's brand of cephalosporin whenever that drug is prescribed, indicating that Template's cephalosporin can be provided to the patient at a very low cost and will generate the greatest profit to Ada Pharmacy. Bill Brewer, a pharmacist with ten years' experience at Ada Pharmacy, is troubled by this decision since Template Pharmaceuticals was recently fined by the Food and Drug Administration for manufacturing infractions, and as yet does not provide laboratory or clinical data on their products to dispensing pharmacists. As Bill patiently explains to a patient why he is using a generic form of cephalosporin, he is distressed when the patient asks, "Is this product as good as the brand-name version?"

**Commentary:** Pharmacists have long presented themselves to the general public as not only experts on drugs but also as convenient and reliable sources for clinical and technical medical information. The two virtues of *candor* and *truthfulness* are highly admired among all health-care professionals and may well be the moral foundation of professional pharmacy practice. This case tests the pharmacist's ability to observe candor and truthfulness in the daily practice of pharmacy. Article IV of the Code of Ethics for Pharmacists speaks of honesty and integrity, recognizing the pharmacist's duty to tell the truth to patients and act with conviction of conscience. At issue in this case may be the extent of disclosure Bill Brewer believes is necessary for discussing the answer to the patient's query. For example, should he discuss how the specific generic manufacturer is selected and the clinical and economic principles used in making the selection? Even though Bill considered this information in making his drug product selection, this sort of information is often beyond the particular needs of the patient. Remember, all that the patient asked was, "Is this product as good as the brand-name version?" An appropriate response could be "Yes" or "No!" Most experienced pharmacists would probably begin with some degree of obfuscation or "benevolent deception" approach: "The federal government has released this for the market so it has got to be good," thus relying on the authority of the government as verification for efficacy. Others may simply say, "We have used this brand for quite a while now and everyone seems pleased with the results." While both responses attempt to avoid direct confrontation with the issue and may be completely truthful, are they the truth? In this case, Bill has another course he may take: "Just a minute, Mr. Lehr is available and he is the best person to answer your question." Shifting decision-making and professional responsibilities to another person may be comforting to Bill, it denies the seriousness of the situation. Eventually, Bill will need to decide whether he will share all available information with his patients in cases such as these and allow them to participate in making the final decision concerning the source of drug.

## Decisions influenced by codes or rules

Some pharmacists prefer to appeal to some external authority, such as a code of ethics, to help them resolve their ethical dilemmas. Unfortunately, as we have noted, some codes of ethics are so general and vague that they are not very useful in resolving specific problems. Relying upon professional etiquette, a series of "gentlemen's agreements"—unwritten, but generally accepted practices which have evolved over the years—can prove even more troublesome. Close business relationships between physicians and pharmacists, for example, are generally considered unethical not only because they raise the specter of financial collusion, but because they might interfere with patients' freedom of choice of health-care providers by creating a temptation to direct patients to a particular provider. In the realm of professional etiquette, this ethical rule has been extended to prohibit one health-care practitioner from recommending another's services. Can a pharmacist in good conscience recommend that a patient consult a certain physician or dentist? What if a patient asks your opinion about a health-care practitioner in whom you have no confidence? Bill Chapman deals with this dilemma in Case 2.3.

### Case 2.3: Conflicts in Professional Etiquette

*"Can you recommend a good physician?"*

Bill Chapman was busy unpacking a drug order when a middle-aged man with distinguished features approached the prescription area. Bill had seen this individual several times in the last month or so and supposed him to be new to the community. As the man neared, Bill introduced himself and asked if he could help. In rapid fashion, the man recounted a long list of medical problems, an equally long list of prescription drugs, and multiple physician encounters. The man not only seemed to know a lot about his drug therapy, but openly questioned the competence of the physicians he had been seeing. "I'm sick and tired of all these quacks!" the man exclaimed. "I've heard good things about Dr. Perkins and his chelation therapy. What's your opinion of him?" Bill was stunned. Dr. Perkins had a long and sordid reputation among pharmacists and physicians alike because of his questionable use of mild electric currents to stimulate weight reduction. Recently, Dr. Perkins had added intravenous ethylenediamine tetraacetic acid (EDTA) infusions for hyperlipidemia and atherosclerosis to his list of questionable practices. Bill had absolutely no confidence in Dr. Perkins, whom he regarded as a charlatan. How should Bill respond to the man's query?

Commentary:  The Code of Ethics for Pharmacists, with its firm foundation on moral principles and virtues, seems to speak directly to this encounter. According to the Code, the patient-pharmacist relationship is covenantal, pledging the pharmacist's commitment to patient welfare as well as honesty and integrity in all professional actions. At the same time, the Code warns that pharmacists respect other health professionals who may differ in the "beliefs and values" of therapeutic care. In this case, Bill Chapman is involved in a situation that is not uncommon in the practice of pharmacy. Pharmacists have cultivated themselves for decades in the image of counselor and information source for the general public, offering their services openly and without reservation. Suddenly, Bill is confronted with an immediate situation in which he has to decide between mollifying this patient with oblique, soothing phrases extolling Dr. Perkins's medical talents or defending his view of Dr. Perkins as a charlatan. This case could be more complex that it seems on the surface. For example, the patient may merely be testing Bill about Dr. Perkins's skills, or may be seeking confirmation and reassurance that seeing Dr. Perkins is in fact the right choice. If Bill decides to reveal his lack of confidence in Dr. Perkins, the patient may develop further aversions and ill-feelings toward medical services, perhaps causing some harm to the himself in the long run. Furthermore, Bill apparently has kept his opinion of Dr. Perkins to himself, not approaching Dr. Perkins and attempting to resolve the awkward situation. This in itself may constitute some form of unethical behavior since patients continue to see Dr. Perkins believing they will receive quality care.

## Decisions influenced by legislation

Pharmacists often must choose between following the letter of the law and providing good professional care. This tension is reflected in most codes of ethics which enjoin pharmacists to always obey the law yet always act in the best interest of the patient. Pharmacists usually resolve requests for unauthorized medication and similar conflicts by a simple benefit-to-risk analysis: Does the benefit the patient is likely to receive from the medication outweigh the risks associated with breaking the law? Would the patient be harmed by the interruption of legitimate long-term or chronic therapy? What standards of practice can pharmacists apply to such benefit-to-risk dilemmas? Case 2.4 provides such a challenge.

### Case 2.4: Conflicts between Legal and Ethical Practice

*"Can you give me a few more pills to hold me over?"*

Late one Saturday evening, Maggie Sanger approached the prescription department at her neighborhood pharmacy, anticipating that her long-time pharmacist and confidant, Jack Meakim, would be on duty. To her surprise there was a new face at the prescription counter. "Hi, I'm George Andrews," the pharmacist smiled in greeting, "Can I help you?" "Where's Jack?" Maggie asked, looking a bit crestfallen. "On vacation for a few days," George replied. "I'm just filling in for him. How can I help you?" he repeated. Maggie explained that her packet of oral contraceptives had fallen out of the medicine chest into a sink full of nylons which she had soaking, ruining the tablets. "I need twelve more birth-control pills to complete my cycle," Maggie added. "Can you give me a few more pills to hold me over?" George notes that Maggie has no refills left on her prescription and is unable to contact her physician for authorization. How should George respond?

**Commentary:** The conflict between legal and ethical pharmacy practice is often the choice between following the letter of the law and observing good professional care. When Maggie asks for "Jack," she seems to imply that George might not be able to take care of the problem. Somehow, the new face is going to cause trouble. Many pharmacists would respond to this situation by dismissing the event as casual, with no hesitancy in offering the needed replacement tablets. Others who are more rule-dominated would explain that Maggie needs to see a physician and obtain a new medication order. What the pharmacist ought to do in this type of case depends heavily on the breadth of personal value system the pharmacist holds, especially if the ethics of care (or the context of the case) form an important part of the system.

## Decisions influenced by personal and professional values

To what extent do our personal value systems influence the decisions we make in practice, particularly when those decisions involve a value component contradictory to our professional values? Our religious beliefs, the social mores we are taught in school, and the behavioral patterns we learn at home all combine to forge a powerful—if sometimes internally inconsistent—set of personal values. When a pharmacist chooses not to work in observance of a religious holiday, no conflict in values exist even though some of his patients may be inconvenienced. To what extent, however, can a pharmacist impose his personal belief system or set of values upon his patients while performing his professional services? Case 2.5 provides a thought-provoking example of this conflict.

### Case 2.5: Conflicts between Value Systems

*"What do you mean, you don't carry condoms?"*

Chuck Ellis was very proud of his new prescription-center pharmacy because it gave him the opportunity to know his patients personally and serve them with the best possible professional care. Moreover, as the owner-manager, Chuck was able to establish all the pharmacy's administrative policies. One new policy Chuck established concerned the selling of condoms. A devout Roman Catholic, Chuck understood the Church's teaching that the selling of condoms was forbidden by moral law as "unjustified proximate material cooperation in moral evil." Chuck had always been troubled when he was asked to sell contraceptive devices by his preceptor, and begged to be excused from this duty. Chuck was also troubled by the rapid spread of AIDS and other sexually-transmitted diseases. Now in charge of his own pharmacy, Chuck decided to make condoms available, but only upon request. In this way, Chuck felt, he could monitor condom sales to his patients, selling them only to those individuals who he felt had a "legitimate" need for them. Tom Malteus, the teenaged son of one of his favorite new customers, came in and congratulated Chuck on his new pharmacy. After some small talk, Tom looked around and asked Chuck where he kept his condoms. Chuck replied that he did not carry condoms. Tom's jaw dropped. "What do you mean, you don't carry condoms?" he asked. How should Chuck respond?

**Commentary:** Value systems conflicts between health professionals and their patients are not restricted to the fringe elements of American society. As seen in this case, the conflict may arise during a common request from a neighborhood individual from a similar culture, adding to the difficulties faced by the pharmacist. Chuck Ellis is now in a position that may be difficult to defend since he apparently is making a value decision concerning contraception that espouses his own religious beliefs and thus is extending his personal convictions to others. Furthermore, he uses a "benevolent deception" approach to avoid providing condoms to the young man. How would the dilemma change if Chuck replied, "Tom, in my opinion you have no legitimate use for condoms, therefore I will not supply them to you?"

## Decisions influenced by economic forces

One of the most troubling problems facing health-care professionals is dealing with patients who cannot afford their services. The temporarily indigent patient who does not qualify for public assistance poses a particularly difficult challenge for pharmacists. Unlike lawyers who accept a certain amount of *pro bono* work with indigent clients as an expression of their professional commitment to society or hospitals that budget a certain amount of "free care" to poor patients in their community, today's pharmacists typically avoid situations that could result in "bad debts." Prior to the enactment of Medicare and Medicaid legislation in the mid-1960s, many independent pharmacists responded to the needs of their indigent patients by opening charge accounts, partially filling prescription orders, or in some cases, giving them the needed medication at no charge. This does not mean that today's pharmacists are devoid of benevolent feelings; many pharmacists have continued these practices and take extra care in counseling poor or elderly patients who may not be able to read or interpret standard patient package inserts. Nevertheless, federal and state "welfare" legislation and the increasing corporatization of pharmacy practice have resulted in a more diffused, collective commitment to the indigent population, diminishing many pharmacists' opportunities to offer their personal services to needy individuals. To what extent can employee pharmacists exercise their professional obligation to be altruistic? Case 2.6 explores this dilemma.

### Case 2.6: Conflicts Arising From Profit Motives

*"I don't have the money for this prescription."*

Young Jack Kidwell's ears are burning. He has just received a lecture from his pharmacist-manager Sam Colcord on the importance of increasing profits in the prescription department. "We're not running a nonprofit public service agency here," Mr. Colcord thundered. "From now on, be sure to collect cash for all private-pay prescriptions that you dispense." A short time later, Jack fills an antibiotic prescription for the six-year-old son of Dottie Dix, a young mother whose husband Jack knows has been laid off at the local auto plant for over six months. Jack explains how Dottie should administer the antibiotic to her son and concludes by mentioning the prescription price. "I don't have the money for this prescription," Dottie replies with downcast eyes. Jack knows the little boy needs the medicine and also knows that a partial dosage regimen will not only not cure his infection, but may actually do some harm by encouraging the development of resistant organisms. He is also mindful of Mr. Colcord's new mandate on collecting cash for all prescriptions and realizes that charging the prescription is not an option. What should Jack do to resolve this conflict?

**Commentary:** The opportunity for pharmacists to provide *pro bono* services is often clouded by the significant costs of maintaining a viable prescription center. Unlike other professions where costs for personal services are the predominant factor for charges, pharmacists are faced with expensive drug products comprising the major part of their professional charges. As the number of employee pharmacists increases, they will need to examine the ethical attitude of their practice environment and decide if the corporate value systems are congruent with their own. Jack Kidwell has only a few choices in serving this patient, each requiring careful consideration and perhaps personal sacrifice. One course would be for Jack to pay for the prescription himself, thereby insuring the proper medication for the little boy and averting difficulties with Mr. Colcord. Such altruistic behavior is not uncommon among pharmacists. Another likely approach may be for Jack to meet with Mr. Colcord and propose to budget a certain amount of total revenues for "beneficence," that is, to serve the kind of patient involved in this case. Such an approach could provide for all members of the practice the opportunity to share in the altruistic act, especially if the budgeted amount is augmented with individual contributions. Article VIII of the Code of Ethics for Pharmacists reminds pharmacists of their responsibility toward the just allocation of health-care resources.

## Concluding Remarks

As we have indicated, pharmacists and other health-care practitioners employ a variety of theories and concepts to solve the ethical dilemmas they face in practice. Whether you choose ethical theories, virtues and values, or codes of ethics to develop your own unique set of values as a foundation for decision-making, we strongly encourage you to employ a logical problem-solving approach—such as the one presented in this chapter—to assist you in making consistent, defensible ethical choices. With practice, ethical decision-making can become one of the most satisfying aspects of your professional practice.

## Study Questions

2.1 Discuss consequentialism, nonconsequentialism, social contract theory, and an ethic of care as these concepts apply to pharmacy practice, giving examples of each. Which concept do you personally prefer, and why?

2.2 The 1981 Code of Ethics of the American Pharmaceutical Association calls upon its members to "never knowingly condone the . . . distributing of drugs . . . that lack therapeutic value." Explain why you would—or would not—sell a questionable patent medicine to a patient upon request.

2.3 Describe, in your own words, the concept of the "virtuous pharmacist." What traits of character would such a pharmacist display in his or her practice?

2.4 Explain the foundation for the American Pharmaceutical Association's 1994 Code of Ethics for Pharmacists. Attempt to resolve any potential conflicts with your personal value system.

## Situations for Analysis

2.1 A pharmacist working at a student health center pharmacy on a large campus refuses to fill a prescription for four oral contraceptive tablets once he realizes that the tablets are intended to be used for "morning-after therapy," explaining that his religious beliefs do not condone abortion. "You may have a right to your religious beliefs," the young woman counters, "but you don't have a right to refuse to fill my prescription."

2.2 A young pharmacist working at a university drug information center receives a query about the availability of a naturally occurring plant drug touted in the lay press as a new and potent cancer cure. The pharmacist believes the drug is very question-able—and probably totally ineffective—therapy and begins to explain her concerns to the caller. "I know everything I need to know about this drug, young lady," the caller replies sweetly. "I just need to know where I can order it." The pharmacist is well aware of the drug's source.

2.3  A young pharmacist settles into his new position at a well-estab-lished pharmacy in an exclusive neighborhood. His supervisor explains that certain cough syrups with small amounts of co-deine (Schedule V preparations) are hidden from open view and should only be sold to "the right kind of customers," adding that "we don't want to attract any undesirable traffic in our store." When the young pharmacist presses for clarification, his super-visor advises him to "tell anybody that doesn't look right that we don't carry those kinds of drugs."

# References

1.  Albert [R.] Jonsen, "Fortresses and Formularies: Drugs, Ethics, and Managed Care," *American Journal of Health System Pharmacists 57*:9 (May 1, 2000), p. 854.
2.  Douglas Waugh, "Social Contracts and Health Care," *Canadian Medi-cal Association Journal 149*:9 (November, 1993), pp. 1320-21. "Within the health care professions we tend to think of objectives as targets we ourselves have chosen for our programs. In the context of the social con-tract, expectations are objectives that have been mutually agreed to by the parties to the contract," Waugh notes. "Society cannot dictate to the health professions any more than the professions can lay down the law to the society they serve." *Ibid.*, p. 1321.
3.  Douglas P. Olson, "Populations Vulnerable to the Ethics of Caring," *Journal of Advanced Nursing 18*:11 (November, 1993), p. 1697. Caring imbues professionals with "the power and motivation to advocate for the patient and to treat the patient with dignity and respect," Olson notes, but cautions that "the ethics of caring provides no guide for de-termining which contextual factors are legitimate ethical guides and which are not." *Ibid.*
4.  Virginia A. Sharpe, "Justice and Care: The Implications of the Kohlberg-Gilligan Debate for Medical Ethics," *Theoretical Medicine 13*:4 (Decem-ber, 1992), p. 296. Sharpe notes that because the care perspective "is attentive to real individuals rather than simply to individuals abstractly conceived, it acknowledges the moral significance of real inequalities that may in fact distinguish us." *Ibid.*, pp. 296-97.
5.  See C. D. Broad, *Five Types of Ethical Theory* (London: Routledge and Kegan Paul, 1930), pp. 206 and 278, cited in Tom L. Beauchamp and James F. Childress, *Principles of Biomedical Ethics*, 3rd ed. (New York

and Oxford: Oxford University Press, 1989), p. 62. The term *consequentialism* gained wide currency as a result of G. E. M. Anscombe's article "Modern Moral Philosophy," *Philosophy 33*:124 (January, 1958), pp. 1-19.

6. Tom L. Beauchamp and James F. Childress, *Principles of Biomedical Ethics*, 5th ed. (New York and Oxford: Oxford University Press, 2001), p. 29. "We do not hold that the merit in an action resides in motive or character alone," they continue. "For example, the physician or nurse who is appropriately motivated to help a patient but who acts incompetently in seeking the desired result does not act in a praiseworthy manner." *Ibid*. For a detailed account of moral virtues and character, see Chapter 2, pp. 26-56, *ibid*.

7. See Paul U. Unschuld, "Confucianism," in *Encyclopedia of Bioethics*, ed. by Warren T. Reich (New York: The Free Press, 1978), Vol. 1, p. 200; and Chauncey D. Leake, ed., *Percival's Medical Ethics* (Baltimore: The Williams & Wilkins Company, 1927), p. 71, cited by Robert M. Veatch, *A Theory of Medical Ethics* (New York: Basic Books, Inc., 1981), p. 64.

8. Joseph W. England, ed., *The First Century of the Philadelphia College of Pharmacy, 1821-1921* (Philadelphia: Philadelphia College of Pharmacy and Science, 1922), pp. 56-57; Edward Parrish, "Ethical Analysis," *Proceedings of the American Pharmaceutical Association 6* (1857), p. 148; and Edward C. Elliott, *The General Report of the Pharmaceutical Survey, 1946-49* (Washington, D.C.: American Council on Education, 1950), p. 4.

9. H. John Baldwin and Kelly T. Alberts, "Detailed Cases and Commentary: Introduction," in *Pharmacy Ethics*, ed. by Mickey Smith, Steven Strauss, H. John Baldwin, and Kelly T. Alberts (New York and London: Pharmaceutical Products Press, 1991), p. 452. They conclude that "to the extent that the pharmacist manifests these traits he or she will have internalized the excellences which are particularly definitional of the pharmaceutical profession." *Ibid*.

10. Sixty-seven percent of Americans rated pharmacists "high" or "very high" in ethical standards, second to nurses, who achieved a 79% rating, the Poll reported in November, 2000. Pharmacists had consistently finished first in the survey until nurses were added to the list in 1999. Darren K. Carlson, "Nurses Remain at Top on Honesty and Ethics Poll," *Gallup Poll Monthly*, No. 422 (November, 2000), pp. 45-48.

11. "Code of Ethics of the American Pharmaceutical Association," *Proceedings of the National Pharmaceutical Convention, Held at Philadelphia, October 6th, 1852* (Philadelphia: Merrihew & Thompson, Printers, 1865), p. 25.

12. "Code of Ethics, American Pharmaceutical Association," *APhA Weekly 15*:40 (October 2, 1976), p. 3. The Code was approved by the membership in December, 1975, and revised in July, 1981, to remove all reference to gender. See "Membership Votes Approval of Changes in Constitution, Bylaws, Code of Ethics," *ibid. 15*:3 (January 17, 1976), p. 1. Also see "Code of Ethics for Pharmacists," approved September, 1993 by the Board of Trustees of the American Pharmaceutical Association and October 27, 1994 by the membership.

13. "Code of Ethics of the American Pharmaceutical Association (Adopted August 17, 1922)," *Journal of the American Pharmaceutical Association 11*:9 (September, 1922), pp. 728-29; and "American Pharmaceutical As-

sociation Code of Ethics" [approved by active and life members, August 1969; amended December, 1975; revised July, 1981], placard issued by the Association. Also see "Code of Ethics for Pharmacists," approved September, 1993 by the Board of Trustees of the American Pharmaceutical Association and October 27, 1994 by the membership.

14.  "Code of Ethics of the American Pharmaceutical Association (Adopted August 17, 1922)," p. 728; and "APhA Code of Ethics," *Journal of the American Pharmaceutical Association NS9*:11 (November, 1969), p. 552. Also see "Code of Ethics for Pharmacists," approved September, 1993 by the Board of Trustees of the American Pharmaceutical Association and October 27, 1994 by the membership.

15.  George H. Kieffer, *Bioethics: A Textbook of Issues* (Reading, Massachusetts: Addison-Wesley Publishing Company, 1979), pp. 317-18. "Medical care must be open equally to all who need it and controlled by those who use it." *Ibid.*, p. 318. The concept of rights and duties is explored in depth by Richard A. Wright in *Human Values in Health Care: The Practice of Ethics* (New York: McGraw-Hill Book Company, 1987), pp. 28-38.

16.  "Pharmacy Patient's Bill of Rights," *U.S. Pharmacist 17*:5 (May, 1992), p. 68. The University of Illinois College of Pharmacy's Hind T. Hatoum identified six external factors that drove the development of the Bill of Rights: the rise of consumerism, an increase in health awareness and education, a desire for information, change in practice settings, a decline of health-care services, and growing patient representation. See Hind T. Hatoum, "Pharmacy's Stake in the Patient's Bill of Rights," *ibid.*, pp. 60-62, 64, 66-67, 88. The NABP Foundation provided a grant to Richard A. Hutchinson and Hatoum to develop a draft of the Bill for its consideration. See Carmen A. Catizone, "NABP's Role in Developing a Bill of Rights," *ibid.*, p. 70; and "NABP Develops Pharmacy Patient's Bill of Rights," *NABP Newsletter 21*:5 (June, 1992), pp. 49, 51.

17.  Norman Daniels, *Just Health Care* (Cambridge: Cambridge University Press, 1985), p. 8. Daniels provides a lucid discussion of the issues involved in the "right" to health care, distinguishing between the right to *health* and the right to *health care*. *Ibid.*, pp. 4-9.

18.  Wright outlines several sources of duties including duties based on religious law, duties based on social rules (including professional codes), and duties derived from reason, logic, or philosophical analysis. See Wright, *Human Values in Health Care* (n. 15), pp. 29-33.

19.  See Daniel B. Smith, Charles Ellis, and Samuel F. Troth, "A Code of Ethics Adopted by the Philadelphia College of Pharmacy," *American Journal of Pharmacy 20*:2 (April, 1848), pp. 148-51; and "Code of Ethics of the American Pharmaceutical Association," *Proceedings of the National Pharmaceutical Convention Held at Philadelphia, October 6th, 1852*, (n. 11), pp. 24-26. Also see Charles H. LaWall, "Pharmaceutical Ethics: A Historical View of the Subject with Examples of Codes Adopted or Suggested at Different Periods, Together with a Suggested Code for Adoption by Present-Day Associations," *Journal of the American Pharmaceutical Association 10*:11 (November, 1921), pp. 898-901.

20.  Robert M. Veatch, *A Theory of Medical Ethics* (New York: Basic Books, Inc., 1981), p. 95. Veatch concludes that "a professional ethics grounded in nothing more than agreement, custom, or vote by a group's members can have no ethical bite." *Ibid.*, p. 97.

21.  [George B. Griffenhagen,] "Our Code of Ethics," *Journal of the Ameri-*

*can Pharmaceutical Association NS3*:2 (February, 1963), p. 65. In 1902, the Code was incorporated in an address by Dr. Frederick Hoffmann commemorating the semicentennial of the Association. In 1915, a committee was appointed to revise the Code, but did not report back to the Association. In 1921, former APhA president and dean of the Philadelphia College of Pharmacy Charles H. LaWall wrote a new and comprehensive Code, which remained the basis for subsequent revisions until 1969. See LaWall, "Pharmaceutical Ethics" (n. 19), p. 901.

22. "Resolutions—1966," *Journal of the American Pharmaceutical Association NS6*:6 (June, 1966), p. 294. "Unprofessional conduct" was defined in the Bylaws of the Association as either a conviction of a law related to pharmacy practice or a violation of the "principles embodied in the Code of Ethics." See Chapter VII, Article II(A), American Pharmaceutical Association Bylaws (adopted May 21, 1969). Four years earlier, the Wisconsin Pharmaceutical Association adopted a similar mechanism for enforcing its new code of ethics, which also included several appended "Statements on Professional Etiquette." The Code was adopted by the Association in October 1962. See Richard S. Strommen, "Professional Activities Report," *The Wisconsin Pharmacist 30*:11 (November, 1962), p. 348; Vernon W. Johnson, "Board of Directors," *ibid.*, p. 346; and "Code of Ethics, Wisconsin Pharmaceutical Association," *ibid., 31*:3 (March, 1963), pp. 72-74.

23. For background reading on this pivotal incident, see "APhA Judicial Board to Proceed Against Nine Code Violators," *APhA Newsletter 9*:5 (March 7, 1970), pp. 1 and 4; Kenneth S. Griswold, "Report of the Judicial Board," *Journal of the American Pharmaceutical Association NS10*:6 (June, 1970), pp. 330-31; "Revco Executive Seeks to Enjoin Michigan Pharmacists' Groups from Further Coercion," news release from Revco D.S., Inc., January 11, 1971, printed in *APhA Newsletter 10*:2 (January 23, 1971), p. 2; "Arnold Executive Seeks to Enjoin Pharmacists' Groups from Further Coercion," news release from Arnold's, Inc., n.d., *ibid.*, pp. 2-3; "NACDS Takes Action to Help Chain Pharmacists," news release from the National Association of Chain Drug Stores, Inc., n.d., *ibid.*, p. 3; "Pharmacy Lawsuits and Association Hearings Canceled," *APhA Newsletter 12*:8 (April 7, 1973), p. 3; and George Griffenhagen, "A History of the APhA Judicial Board and Its Relationship to the APhA Code of Ethics," unpublished manuscript, December 1, 1992, 8 pp. For a full account of the history and development of the APhA Code of Ethics, see Robert A. Buerki, "The Historical Development of an Ethic for American Pharmacy," *Pharmacy in History 39*:2 (1997), pp. 54-72.

24. See David B. Brushwood, "Grounds for Revocation or Suspension of a Pharmacist's License," *American Pharmacy NS22*:11 (November, 1982), p. 574; and Richard R. Abood, "Discretionary Justice and State Boards of Pharmacy," *Contemporary Pharmacy Practice 5*:4 (Fall, 1982), p. 252.

25. In 1969, for example, APhA reaffirmed its policy opposing placement of consumers on professional boards, noting that "members of the general public have no proper place on regulatory boards dealing with highly complex and technical professional matters." Three years later, however, the APhA reversed its policy, encouraging state pharmaceutical associations to "actively seek appointment of lay representatives of the public to their respective boards of pharmacy." See Donald A. Dee, "[Report of Committee on] Legislation," *Journal of the American Pharma-*

*ceutical Association NS9*:7 (July, 1969), p. 349; and "House of Delegates—1972," *ibid. NS12*:6 (June, 1972), p. 281.

26. See Wright, *Human Values in Health Care* (n. 15), pp. 44-63; and Jack Justice, "Objectivity & Critical Thinking to Resolve Ethical Dilemmas in Pharmacy Practice," *Journal of Social and Administrative Pharmacy* 7:2 (1990), pp. 93-98.

27. Kieffer, *Bioethics* (n. 15), p. 48. Kieffer recommends stating the ethical problem as a question that must be answered in terms of a *value object*, an "object about which a value decision must be made."

28. In 1989, for example, Dr. James C. Burt surrendered his license to the Ohio State Medical Board, which was investigating him on the charge that he unnecessarily performed genital surgery on women under the pretense that it increased sexual satisfaction. Many patients suffered sexual dysfunction, infection, and pain from the so-called "love surgery." Two years later a Dayton, Ohio jury awarded Janet Phillips $5 million in damages based on her claim that Dr. Burt maimed her by reconstructing her vagina without her permission; nineteen similar claims were later dismissed. See "Physician Charged Over 'Love Surgery' Surrenders License," *New York Times*, January 27, 1989, Sec. A, p. 13; "$5 Million Awarded to Woman Who Said Doctor Maimed Her," *ibid.*, June 22, 1991, Sec. A, p. 9; and "Suits Against Ex-Gynecologist Are Rejected," *ibid.*, September 8, 1991, Sec. 1, p. 21.

# Suggested Readings

Hauerwas, Stanley. *Naming the Silences: God, Medicine, and the Problem of Suffering*. Grand Rapids, Michigan: William B. Eerdmans Publishing Company, 1990.

Jonsen, Albert R., ed. "The Birth of Bioethics." Special Supplement, *Hastings Center Report 23*:6 (November- December, 1993), pp. S1-S16.

"Solemn Oath of a Physician of Russia." *Kennedy Institute of Ethics Journal 3*:4 (December, 1993), p. 419.

Veatch, Robert M., and Haddad, Amy [M.]. *Case Studies in Pharmacy Ethics*. New York: Oxford University Press, 1999.

Verhey, Allen, and Lammers, Stephen E., eds. *Theological Voices in Medical Ethics*. Grand Rapids, Michigan: William B. Eerdmans Publishing Company, 1993.

# CHAPTER 3

# THE PHARMACIST-PATIENT RELATIONSHIP

Authors in the fields of medicine, nursing, and bioethics have presented dramatic descriptions of the physician-patient and the nurse-patient relationship.[1] These depictions are often grounded in moral principles such as "justice," "beneficence," or "autonomy," as well as general theories of moral philosophy. In their text *Principles of Biomedical Ethics*, Beauchamp and Childress focus more clearly on the relationship between health professionals and their patients, specifically on the meaning of "faithfulness" of one human to another.[2] William F. May shifts the focus of this rather contractual relationship to embrace the frankly theological concept of a solemn "covenant" that exists between health professionals and their patients, based upon the practitioners' sense of indebtedness toward a society which permits them to perform their professional function.[3] Scholars have rarely extended this analysis to the profession of pharmacy or explored the underlying nature of the pharmacist-patient relationship. The covenantal nature of the 1994 Code of Ethics for Pharmacists, coupled with the acceptance of the practice philosophy of pharmaceutical care, which is also explained in terms of a convenantal relationship, may bring the profession of pharmacy closer to this ideal.

While some pharmacists might feel uncomfortable using the term "covenant" to describe their everyday relationships with their patients, this tension underscores the rather recent shift in professional development described in the last chapter, a shift that moved "druggists" from waiting on their "customers" to "pharmacists" serving their "patients." In moving toward a description of the pharmacist-patient relationship, we must go beyond the functional definition of pharmacy practice, which is bounded by the safe, accurate, and legal distribution of dangerous drugs toward a more patient-centered practice that relies upon the ability of pharmacists to establish an authentic interpersonal relationship with their patients.

71

This relationship includes not only the counseling function that attends the dispensing of prescription and nonprescription medication, but also a variety of professional activities which allows the pharmacist to emerge as a proactive advocate for "high-level wellness," a term that embraces both health maintenance and life-style considerations. In this regard, Brody goes so far as to suggest that health-care practitioners recognize, respect, and coordinate their treatment plans with their patients' "life plans," those idiosyncratic activities that can compromise so-called "rational" medical care.[4] For example, an obese patient may place a higher value upon gourmet dining than upon the promise of an extended life a recommended bland diet might offer, "rational" as the latter course of action might seem to his physician.

### The nature of the pharmacist-patient relationship

Expanding the concept of the pharmacist-patient relationship beyond the distributive function carries with it an obligation to treat even casual encounters with pharmacy patrons with the duty one ordinarily associates with physicians and their relationships with their patients. This concept is often complicated by low—perhaps misunderstood—public expectations for pharmaceutical services beyond the minimal distributive function. Once adopted, this higher level of professional responsibility emerges as a legally recognized standard of practice that does not necessarily require even tacit acceptance on the part of patients. In the past, the profession of pharmacy has proclaimed its adherence to this higher calling without reflecting sufficiently upon the serious ethical consequences that can flow from enhanced patient-care services.

**The fiduciary aspect of the relationship.** Trust is inherent in the relationship between health-care professionals and their patients. This condition is a reflection of the system of licensure that is imposed by society, which permits patients to place their most intimate thoughts as well as their bodies in the hands of professionals whose competency they cannot easily judge. In contrast to the practice of medicine and nursing, which is characterized by direct patient contact, the pharmacist often purposely fills prescription orders in seclusion or partially shielded from the patient's watchful eyes, requiring even greater faith in the pharmacist's competence, a faith that is reflected in recent public opinion polls.[5] Whether this high regard for pharmacists is actually warranted or merely an artifact of public glimpses of the rather mysterious "act" of pharmacy remains an open question. As the practice of pharmacy expands to include more intense interpersonal encounters, this comforting public trust will be increasingly challenged as patients have expanded opportunities to scrutinize and evaluate the services they receive.

**The voluntary aspect of the relationship.** In its simplest form, the pharmacist-patient relationship begins when a patient presents a pharmacist with a request for a professional service, a voluntary act upon which a trusting relationship is grounded. This relationship is thus *patient-initiated*, offering the pharmacist the *opportunity* to provide professional service. This distinction is often lost in the heat of "freedom of choice" debates that usually hinge upon the "unprofessional" practice of physicians, insurance companies, and other third parties who direct patients to selected pharmacists with whom they have established a contractual arrangement. Patients normally select their pharmacists and their attendant array of professional services in a highly visible, straightforward manner. Even in the rigid confines of an acute-care hospital, patients may choose to consult with a pharmacist who is more closely attuned to their needs. An appreciation of the voluntary nature of the pharmacist-patient relationship is necessary to properly understand the covenantal character of this relationship.

**The covenantal aspect of the relationship.** According to May, a covenantal relationship is based upon the concepts of indebtedness and responsiveness. The work of a health professional begins with a response to a patient's request for assistance or care. The patient thus provides the "gift" of a personal sanction to the health practitioner to initiate professional service, thereby assuring the need for patient involvement in all aspects of pharmaceutical care. This "gift" creates a sense of indebtedness or gratitude on the part of the practitioner, which provides him with an opportunity to perform his professional functions.[6] Implicit in this covenant is the commitment to not only maintain a high quality of technical skill but also to safeguard patients from untoward actions related to their drug therapy. In addition, pharmacists accept the covenantal obligation to dutifully observe the personal rights of their patients and thereby manifest their respect for their human dignity.[7] The covenantal aspect of the pharmacist-patient relationship thus goes far beyond any legal or contractual relationship they may have established in other contexts.

### The complexity of the pharmacist-patient relationship

Whereas the relationship between the physician and his patient has evolved over the past several decades to include increasingly complex technical and clinical functions, the basic service component of this relationship continues to be patient care and the eradication of disease. In contrast, the professional function of pharmacists during this same period has slowly evolved from a primarily distributive function in a mercantile setting to an expanding consultative function in an increasingly clinical setting. Unfortunately, the public often neither understands nor appreciates the advantages of pharmaceutical care, and seems content to purchase their prescription drugs as needed without requesting the expanded service many pharmacists now offer. This disparity between professional needs and public expectations creates serious functional stresses that often frustrate pharmacists who wish to provide their patients with the highest level of professional care.

**The functional complexity of the relationship.** The pharmacist-patient relationship is often exacerbated by the environment that surrounds this relationship. In many cases, pharmacists attempt to perform their professional functions in an isolated environment, far removed from both their patients and the medical records they need to provide pharmaceutical care. While this is becoming less of an issue in institutional settings, it remains as a challenge to community pharmacists who continue to provide the vast majority of pharmaceutical services to ambulatory patients. Unfortunately, the community pharmacists who attempt to establish strong and supportive relationships with their patients often do so without the benefit of access to sufficient clinical information. Patients who choose their pharmaceutical services primarily on the basis of convenience further compromise the effectiveness of professional consultation that the continuity of pharmaceutical care offers. Until such time as an adequate information network is developed, pharmacists must rely upon their interpersonal communication skills to identify and resolve the therapeutic problems faced by their patients.[8]

**The dimensional complexity of the relationship.** The pharmacist-patient relationship is imbedded within the classic physician-pharmacist-patient triad. Whether viewed as "customers," "consumers," or "patients," pharmacists instinctively emphasize their relationships with their clientele, particularly as these relationships

can affect their income. "The hallmark of community pharmacy is
the patient-pharmacist relationship," a Texas pharmacist emphasized. "All pharmacists should take the time to learn about their
patients and their individual needs."[9] This emphasis upon the economic aspects of pharmacy practice serves as an especially troublesome constraint to pharmacists who may wish to develop a covenant with their patients, but who fear they cannot "afford" to do
so in an increasingly competitive health-care marketplace. This
emphasis upon economics can also overshadow the relationship between the pharmacist and the prescribing physician, especially if
the pharmacist views the physician only as a source of prescription
orders or "business." Moreover, an economically driven model of
professional practice often places the pharmacist in a subservient
position to the physician and undermines the footing upon which
value-based pharmacist-physician and pharmacist-patient relationships depend. As increasingly greater numbers of patients seek
their medical and pharmaceutical services from managed health-
care systems in which both physicians and pharmacists are employed as collegial members of a health-care team, the traditional
reliance upon creating and maintaining economic notions of "good
will" will become subordinated to issues which maximize improved
patient care.

## The Moral Basis of the Pharmacist-Patient Relationship

Even at the most elemental, distributive level of pharmacy practice, pharmacists make decisions that affect their patients—moral
decisions which affect human purposes. Recall that the *General Report of the Pharmaceutical Survey* (1950) concluded that "the outstanding factor determining the future of the profession of pharmacy is fundamentally moral in nature."[10] More recently,
Pellegrino and Thomasma elegantly encapsulated the moral dimension to the pharmacist-patient relationship when they declared
that "any act which applies knowledge to persons involves values
and consequently falls into the moral realm."[11] While some pharmacists may feel uncomfortable using the term "moral" to describe
their everyday behavior toward their patients, most would agree
that they often make professional decisions based upon what is
"good" for the patient, rather than upon what may be scientifically
or even legally "correct." It is in this context that the word

"moral" may be properly applied to the pharmacist-patient relationship and the moral principles upon which this relationship depends.

## Moral principles affecting the relationship

Framers of the earliest codes of professional medical practice presumed that their codes would reflect their patients' best interests. Based upon the ancient Hippocratic principle of doing good and avoiding evil, these codes enjoined medical practitioners to always behave in a manner that would benefit their patients. Whereas physicians traditionally look to the ancient Hippocratic Oath as their source of moral guidance, pharmacists ordinarily look to their professional associations to provide guidelines for good professional practice, generally in the form of a code of ethics. Until recently, however, most of these codes merely listed acts or relationships traditionally thought to be "nonprofessional" or "unethical" without solidly grounding them in moral principles.

In the years following World War II, this somewhat restrictive system of codified ethics has been characterized as being rather exclusive and self-serving. For example, in 1985, pharmacist and ethicist Robert M. Veatch challenged America's pharmacists to "respond to the critical questions of the day," especially as they moved "beyond the traditional conception of our profession."[12] Veatch argued persuasively that a wide range of moral principles must be considered in developing a more comprehensive ethic for the contemporary practice of pharmacy. Such principles include *beneficence, nonmaleficence, justice,* and *autonomy.**

**Beneficence.** The principle of beneficence is deeply rooted in the fabric of health care. In the context of patient care, *health-care practitioners display beneficence when they act for the good of the patient.* For example, practitioners can prevent their patients from harm, remove harmful conditions, and provide positive health-care benefits to their patients. While these "good acts" reflect the Hippocratic principle of beneficence, they may force the practitioner to compromise other strongly held values. Pharmacists often knowingly break the letter of the law to provide doses of medica-

---

*This discussion is adopted from Robert A. Buerki and Louis D. Vottero, "Ethics," Chapter 11 in *Pharmacy Practice: Social and Behavioral Aspects,* 3rd ed., edited by Albert I. Wertheimer and Mickey C. Smith (Baltimore, Maryland: University Park Press, 1989), pp. 333-35.

tion that they believe are essential for their patients' well-being. Like the Biblical Samaritan who went out of his way to help a stranger, today's proactive pharmacist seeking to fully implement pharmaceutical care brings to bear the full power of the professional duty to observe beneficence.

**Nonmaleficence.** The 1969 Code of Ethics of the American Pharmaceutical Association required the pharmacist to "never knowingly condone the dispensing . . . of drugs . . . that lack therapeutic value."[13] This statement is the closest the Code came to referring to the principle of nonmaleficence. *Health practitioners display nonmaleficence when they act to prevent, or at least not inflict, evil or harm upon their patients.* William K. Frankena sees nonmaleficence as the lowest level of beneficence, in the sense that doing no harm is the least intrusive of a wide spectrum of beneficent acts.[14] The concept of nonmaleficence is the essence of the Hippocratic Oath, embodied in the injunction *primum non nocere*— "first, do no harm." Centuries later, Edward Parrish asked, "How far is it the duty of the pharmaceutist, in the sale of stimulant and narcotic agents, to interfere for the prevention of their intemperate use?"[15] This 1857 admonition anticipates the dilemma presented to pharmacists today by patients who seek assistance in obtaining drugs of unknown or doubtful efficacy—or those drugs which are efficacious, but are used inappropriately, such as psychoactive drugs which have a high addictive potential when used in long-term therapy. Some pharmacists choose not to carry such unproven drugs, and also may not stock items such as homeopathic medications, alcoholic beverages, or tobacco, thus extending the concept of nonmaleficence to a logical extreme.

**Justice.** The principle of justice, as applied to health care, refers to *the strategy by which health practitioners allocate goods and services to their patients in an equitable manner.* Such a strategy may include social, economic, and religious issues, and may be further complicated by competing theories of moral philosophy.[16] Classroom discussions of justice invariably center on such issues as how hospital ethics committees select patients to receive scarce and expensive health-care resources, such as access to a kidney dialysis machine. In contrast, the allocation of professional services to an ever-increasing aged population provides a less dramatic, but equally pressing example of the need for practitioners to apply the principle of justice to their patients. Patients have the right to be treated fairly in their dealings with all health-care practitioners.

Pharmacists often extend credit or make other special arrangements to their marginally indigent patients, allowing them access to their frequently expensive maintenance drugs. The principle of justice applies to the pharmacist's relationships with patients at all levels of the socioeconomic spectrum, ranging from the very wealthy to those receiving public assistance. In 1857, Parrish asked if it was

morally right for a pharmaceutist who has the confidence of the poor and ignorant of his neighborhood, to take indiscriminately their hard earnings in exchange for the costly and often worse than useless medicines, which, through the public press are plausibly and insidiously recommended to them?[17]

Today, for pharmacists to selectively deny professional services to Medicaid recipients or other "undesirable" patients based solely upon their inability to pay violates the principle of justice. In the late 1970s, groups of pharmacists around the country refused to fill Medicaid prescriptions in protest against low reimbursement fee schedules, burdensome paperwork, and delays in receiving payment. Seymour Banner and Carol Levine argue that by agreeing to participate in the Medicaid program, "pharmacists have accepted a social obligation to serve a group of clients that society has decided has a right to certain medical services at public expense," concluding that "temporary withdrawal of services for a particular economic goal violates a public trust."[18] Pharmacists have a positive duty to treat all their patients in a just and equitable manner, regardless of their appearance, ability to pay, level of education, or literacy.

**Autonomy.** Many moral philosophers consider the principle of respect for autonomy to be paramount in formulating a contemporary code of professional conduct. The beneficence-based Hippocratic Oath reflected traditional attitudes toward medical care in the sense that physicians were to work for the benefit of the sick according to their "ability and judgment" without necessarily including patients in the decision-making process surrounding their therapy. Unfortunately, many practitioners are still guided by the traditional paternalistic view that they know what is in the best interest of their patients. Autonomous patients have the right to decided what—if any—medical treatment they will accept, based upon advice offered by their health practitioners. Thus, *pharmacists and physicians respect the autonomy of their patients by allowing them to exercise their right of therapeutic self-determination.* The ethical value associated with this principle is expressed through the patient's right to *informed consent*, the knowledge base upon which a patient may rationally choose or refuse treatment.

Beauchamp and Childress argue that patients must not only have access to a knowledge base, but be able to deal with the knowledge in a rational manner.[19] Many pharmacists unintentionally violate this right by assuming that their patients are not interested in or would not understand the technical information associated with their prescription medication. Other pharmacists compromise this right by assuming that providing a *Physicians' Desk Reference* for their patients to peruse provides ample opportunities for their informed consent. In the late 1970s, organized medicine and pharmacy resisted the proposed inclusion of patient package inserts with all prescription drugs dispensed on the basis of increased cost and decreased efficiency in the dispensing process rather than on the right of patients to have access to complete and relevant printed information concerning their medications. The frequent patient query, "What's this drug used for?" provides the proactive pharmacist an opportunity not only to reinforce the physician's often sketchy therapeutic directions, but also to confirm whether or not the patient in fact has enough knowledge to consent in an informed manner to the therapy prescribed. Today, professional organizations and individual practitioners alike increasingly promote proactive, professional behaviors which tend to enhance their patients' autonomy. As the professional roles encompassed within the practice philosophy of pharmaceutical care continue to evolve, the duty to respect the autonomy of patients to choose to use—or not use—their prescribed drugs in an informed manner may provide pharmacists with their most difficult ethical challenge.

## Observing faithfulness in the relationship

The primal grounding for the pharmacist-patient relationship is the concept of faithfulness, usually expressed in terms of *fidelity*. While philosophers may argue about whether or not fidelity is a separate moral principle or merely an aspect of another more encompassing moral principle, they usually agree that health practitioners and their patients enter into a contractual, even covenantal, relationship in which promise-keeping—or fidelity—is an integral part. Pharmacists and physicians cultivate their patient relationships in a manner that invites the trust of their patients by promising to act in their best interests. Patients who trust their pharmacists implicitly also become extremely vulnerable to the consequences of the health-care decisions made on their behalf. When pharmacists make these decisions on other criteria, they break this promise and thus weaken the trust relationship. *To keep the promise to act in the patient's best interest is to practice fidelity within the pharmacist-patient relationship.* Two of the most important duties associated with the principle of fidelity are *veracity* and *confidentiality.* Indeed, to tell the truth and to observe the confidence of the patient may well be the essential nexus of the pharmacist-patient relationship.

**Veracity.** In the simplest terms, *veracity is the duty to tell the truth and not to lie or to deceive others.* While beguilingly simple and outwardly appealing, the duty to always tell the truth may not be absolute. Does the duty of veracity require pharmacists to tell their patients "the truth, the whole truth, and nothing but the truth," only part of the truth, or just that portion of the truth that they can—or should—"understand?" The answer to these questions often is, "It depends." Placebo therapy is a case in point: physicians may choose to treat their patients with an inert substance or with subtherapeutic doses of active agents in order to prompt a nonpharmacological response. In so doing, these physicians apparently deceive their patients to achieve a greater good. Unless pharmacists are aware of the physicians' therapeutic intent in prescribing placebos, they may inadvertently undermine this therapy by responding frankly and truthfully to patients' questions about the effectiveness of their medication.

By the same token, patients often ask their pharmacist to help them judge whether their physician is a "good doctor." The traditional ethical injunction against speaking ill of one's colleagues usually resulted in pharmacists mumbling a few hasty words of assurance, even if they felt uneasy about a physician's qualifications. Veatch declares that such self-serving protectionism "cannot be defended in the present moral climate with its independent principle of veracity."[20] The presumed threat of lost prescription revenue from alienated physicians has made uncompromised veracity a difficult moral tenet for entrepreneurial community pharmacists to reconcile in their daily practice. As a growing cadre of employee pharmacists shifts their attention to embrace concepts of pharmaceutical care, the ideal of true veracity in health care may be more completely realized.

**Confidentiality.** Whereas pharmacists may encounter some difficulty in resolving situations that involve telling their patients the unvarnished truth, maintaining prescription records and their therapeutic indications in close confidence is a time-honored ethical tradition. The 1922 Code of Ethics of the American Pharmaceutical Association implored the pharmacist to "consider the knowledge which he gains of the ailments of his patrons and their confidences . . . as entrusted to his honor," and to "never divulge such facts unless compelled to do so by law." Interestingly, the 1969 Association Code allowed the pharmacist to break patient confidence when "the best interest of the patient requires" such a breach.[21] This exception to the principle of confidentiality was based upon the traditional commitment to patient beneficence, and often resulted in paternalistic behavior as pharmacists attempted to judge the circumstances under which their patients' "best interests" required a breach of confidence. Veatch saw this exception as exceedingly vague and subject to overly broad interpretation. He proposed that the Association embrace a standard similar to that adopted by the American Medical Association, which permits exceptions to the principle only when disclosure of patient information might prevent "serious bodily harm to another person," especially when the "patient is likely to carry out the threat."[22] The 1994 Code of Ethics for Pharmacists partially overcomes Veatch's objections by stating that "a pharmacist promotes the good of every patient in a caring, compassionate, and confidential manner," a unqualified standard that allows pharmacists to exercise their professional judgment in such cases.[23]

While pharmacists are rarely confronted with such dramatic, life-threatening choices, they should remember that confidentiality is an integral part of every patient encounter and also extends to knowledge of their patients' life styles. For example, a pharmacist who sells a package of condoms to the adolescent daughter of a close friend may experience conflict, especially when the friend takes the pharmacist aside and boasts of his daughter's innocent ways. Thus, while the issue of confidentiality in pharmacist-patient relationships may appear simple and straightforward, they can be deceptively complex and potentially troublesome.

## Incorporating other patient-centered values

Current societal value systems reflect a shift away from the traditional strong emphasis on moral rules and ethical principles, resulting in an increased dependence on other values, such as character and virtue. In his analysis of the shift in moral values over time, Daniel Callahan envisioned "a resurgence in social ethics and an emphasis on community," and warned that "an emphasis on rules has the ironic result of often minimizing ethical values, isolating the individual from the community."[24] In moving beyond a principle-based theory toward a virtue-based theory, health-care practitioners should consider using ideals and virtues as guiding principles for shaping their patient relationships. Such personal introspections may lead practitioners to shift the focus of their ethical judgments from considering alternative outcomes of impersonal clinical treatments to the guiding influence of their own personal value system, a system which ordinarily incorporates such human characteristics as ideals and virtues.

**Ideals.** Basic human values such as ideals and virtues beg for definition, but are more easily described by example. Some surgeons are notorious for their impersonal treatment of their patients, and often refer to them as cases—"the gall bladder in 425"— rather than as individuals. Pharmacists can be described as "living up to ideals" by simply being more understanding or considerate to their difficult patients. In a more general sense, *actions prompted by ideals may be considered as conduct which is morally optional, but meritorious or praiseworthy.* The value of ideals may be less forceful than morals in guiding personal behavior, but ignoring the power of ideals may result in feelings of guilt or shame. The pharmacist motivated by ideals treats all patients equally without regard for their appearance, socioeconomic level, or personal demeanor.

**Virtues.** If ideals can be identified with personal standards, *virtues may be identified with the praiseworthy behavior of good or virtuous individuals.* Unfortunately, contemporary society seems to have lost a consensus regarding what constitutes virtuous behavior. "There is no vantage point from which to judge what is right and good," Pellegrino and Thomasma point out. "Virtues becomes confused with conformity to the conventions of social and institutional life." The accolades, they add, go to "those who get along and get ahead."[25] In professional practice, the pharmacist displays not only those virtues that are based upon moral reasoning and theory, but also such value-based virtues as integrity, modesty, and compassion. For example, the pharmacist who supplies prescription medication to a patient in a medical emergency without regard to possible legal consequences does so more out of a sense of human compassion than ethical duty or moral obligation. In the final analysis, virtue may be the quintessential basis for judging ethical behavior in pharmacy practice.

## Conflicts among Role Obligations

In Chapter 2, we traced the development of the pharmacist's professional functions, including the dramatic shift from a predominantly product-centered practice to one in which patient concerns prevail. This shift in practice carries with it a new set of professional expectations and obligations that can produce serious role conflicts and ethical dilemmas. Educator Robert G. Mrtek attributes these conflicts to the persistence of a double paradigm in pharmacy practice: an older technical paradigm in which practice roles were defined in terms of pharmacists distributing drugs in a safe and accurate manner, and a newer clinical paradigm in which practice roles are described in terms of pharmacists solving patient-related therapy problems, often in consultation with other health-care practitioners.[26] These two paradigms coexist uncomfortably in the contemporary practice of pharmacy, and can often result in serious conflicts of values between older and younger pharmacists. In terms of patient consultation, for example, pharmacists operating under the older, passive paradigm discussed nothing substantive with their patients, and often circumvented such discussions by referring all but the most trivial patient questions to the physician. Pharmacists operating under the contemporary active paradigm of pharmaceutical care embrace not only a positive mandate to counsel patients, but also a commitment to rational drug therapy, ensuring that medications are used safely, effectively, and with the least possible expenditure of scarce resources.

## Maintaining patient faithfulness

Pharmacists are often confronted by situations which test their ability to deal with sensitive patient-care information. In many instances, the duty to respect the patient's confidences is compromised by pressures from authority figures who may not share the pharmacists' value systems. The following exercises are designed to assist the responsible pharmacist to internalize the concept of fidelity and apply it consistently without becoming trapped in the quagmire of situational ethics.*

---

*"Situational ethics" or "quandary ethics" refers to narrowly applying one or more moral principles to a discrete dilemma, thus ignoring larger issues and their possible consequences.

### Case 3.1: Loyalty to Patient Care

*"Did the patient tell you anything else?"*

Hank Kiersted, a senior pharmacy student in a strenuous clinical pharmacy program, is assigned to a small teaching hospital. His clinical clerkship requires him to prepare detailed drug histories and maintain critical treatment files on each of his patients. One of his patients, an elderly female, becomes especially talkative during his drug history interview, revealing intensely personal—if somewhat irrelevant—information about herself. "Why, even the doctor doesn't know some of these things," she confides. As Hank completes his assignment, he becomes increasingly concerned about including this sensitive information, even though he knows his report is being graded on the basis of completeness. He decides to omit the sensitive information because he feels it compromises the patient's confidence in him and does not contribute to her care. As a result, his report is rather sketchy. During recitation, his clinical instructor inquires, "Did the patient tell you anything else?" How should Hank respond and why? How absolute is the pharmacist's loyalty to the patient?

**Commentary:** Evolving practices within the profession of pharmacy are moving pharmacists closer and closer to the patient, eventually producing a greater exposure to information that is critically more sensitive and confidential. Hank Kiersted is now confronted with a personal challenge that is not uncommon to contemporary pharmacy practice; he must choose between the duty to respect the confidence of the patient and the need to satisfy the demands of his clinical instructor. By remaining silent to the question of further information Hank may jeopardize his course evaluation or otherwise look bad to the instructor. Hank sees the situation as pitting the possibility of personal gain against the right of the patient for confidentiality. Many courses of action are available for Hank, each with its own merits and unwanted consequences. He could speak frankly to his instructor, explaining carefully about his need to respect the confidences placed upon him by the patient. He also could discuss the matter with the patient, seeking permission to release all pertinent information. Emerging practice roles in pharmacy are presenting additional moral and ethical concerns. As pharmaceutical education attempts to support the pharmaceutical care philosophy of practice by shifting teaching venues from traditional classroom and practice laboratories to actual medical practice sites, more intense ethical dilemmas will present themselves. Some of the more troubling of these dilemmas are those where the pharmacy student—or practicing pharmacist—face the test of competing loyalties. In this case, Hank is tempted by his clinical instructor to disclose certain information that is apparently to be held in confidence—or information that was not provided to the attending physician by the patient. Hank has a number of conflicts to examine and resolve, including the need for the "critical treatment file" to be as complete as possible, the advisability of presenting the information to the attending physician, whether to "shade the truth" to the clinical instructor, or perform as a true advocate for the patient and refrain from divulging any of the "intensely personal" information.

### Case 3.2: Observing Employment Policies

*"Miss Cooper is our best customer. Refill it!"*

As a pharmacy intern, Beth Marshall tries to apply the concepts she learns in the classroom, especially as they relate to patient care. Miss Cooper, a middle-aged patient with chronic asthma and a fiery temper, approaches with an empty inhaler canister and curtly requests a refill, adding "be quick about it!" In reviewing her patient profile, Beth notes that Miss Cooper has been requesting her refills on an increasingly frequent basis, which could compromise her therapy. Beth explains that she cannot refill her inhaler in good conscience until the following week. Miss Cooper complains loudly, demanding to speak to Mr. Moore, her old friend and Beth's boss. Mr. Moore angrily turns to Beth and barks, "Miss Cooper is one of our best customers. Refill it!" Beth feels Mr. Moore's order is not justified on the basis of good patient care, but is confused. What should Beth do and why? How does the situation change if the prescription is authorized to be refilled "prn?"

Commentary: The issue of fidelity to one's professional practice standards is encountered daily, often involving authority figures who attempt to influence or alter these personally held standards. Student pharmacists are deeply influenced by preceptors and need to be able to sort out the underlying foundation for deciding a course of action in a situation such as Beth Marshall's. Beth is involved in a conflict that pits the idealism of a student with the realities of a typical patient service request, the kind of situation pharmaceutical care is designed to avert. Furthermore, she has broadened the conflict by responding directly to the patient before she sought the advice of her preceptor. The preceptor also adds intensity to the moment by ordering immediate action, without the benefit of talking with Beth. Beth has grounds to justify her refusal to provide medications that she considers excessive and harmful on appeal to the Code of Ethics for Pharmacists, or perhaps her belief and commitment to the principle of nonmaleficence.

## Restricting professional services

Sometimes structural and process components can interfere with the delivery of good professional services by even the most conscientious pharmacist. These components can include both physical structures, such as high prescription counters, and managerial barriers, such as policies that restrict or preclude professional services. Other restrictions in professional services may arise from the market-driven economic model under which patients receive their pharmacy services from a variety of convenient outlets or from one designated provider.

### Case 3.3: Curtailing Counseling Services

*"Sorry, the pharmacist can't speak with you."*

As a newly registered pharmacist, Bill Procter is aware of the importance of good patient counseling. He always represents himself to the patient in a forthright and professional manner, and lives with the expectation that his practice as a pharmacist will be a matter of self-selected prerogatives that sustain his vision of the pharmacist-patient relationship. Recently, his nonpharmacist supervisor told him to "forget all that clinical stuff and try to increase your productivity." Bill is especially dumbfounded one day when a patient who has just received a prescription that Bill has completed asks to see the pharmacist. His supervisor replies, "Sorry, the pharmacist can't speak with you." What response should Bill make to both patient and supervisor? Should he seek a different position? How does the situation change if the supervisor is also a pharmacist?

**Commentary:** Earlier codes of ethics for pharmacy provided a specific proscription against practicing under terms or conditions that interfered or impaired the proper exercise of professional judgment and skill. The 1994 Code of Ethics for Pharmacists shifts away from such proscriptive statements, relying instead on broad statements of virtue and covenental significance. Interference from the practice environment as presented in this case must now be seen from the covenental relationship foundation. Regardless of what route Bill Procter takes in resolving this dilemma he will face conflict and ultimately must decide the degree of risk he is willing to undertake. By disregarding the "interference" of his supervisor and directly approaching the patient he places his position in jeopardy. He could lose his position, but he would certainly be stating his conviction of responsibility directly to the patient. Resolution of this and similar dilemmas will require Bill to balance the patient's needs and rights with the realities presented by his practice environment.

### Case 3.4: Managing Conflicting Services

*"Can I take this drug with my mail-order prescription?"*

Mrs. Pinkham, a long-time customer of the Safeway Pharmacy, is apprehensive as she approaches the prescription counter. She recently retired after thirty years of teaching English at the local high school, and now is trying to make personal adjustments to the many changes that seem to be occurring in her life. Her thoughts are dominated by economic concerns—increasing rent payments, rising food costs, and high utility bills. The sudden onset of serious high blood pressure presents her with yet another financial crisis. Her pharmacist and former student, Bill Gordon, was not pleased when he found out that Mrs. Pinkham's high-blood-pressure medications were being provided through a mail-order prescription service located in a large eastern city. Her retirement system provides this service, and it would be financially impossible for her to not take advantage of this service. Today, Mrs. Pinkham has a cold and needs some kind of relief. After selecting her favorite nonprescription product she is confused with the many statements that are printed in small type on the package. She approaches Bill and asks him, "Can I take this with my mail-order prescription?" What is the nature of Bill's duty to counsel Mrs. Pinkham, if any? Does Bill's duty extend to other pharmacists' patients?

Commentary: Personal decisions by pharmacists to restrict their services to specific individuals, or to broadly exclude stereotypes such as those with low income, cast an onus on the entire profession. The 1994 Code of Ethics for Pharmacists speaks about "the good of every patient" and to the need to respect the "personal and cultural differences among patients." Individual actions taken with patients such as Mrs. Pinkham will reveal the depth of commitment pharmacists have to this admirable goal. Bill Gordon is faced with the opportunity to demonstrate not only his personal value system but also his vision of the nature of his profession. If he is concerned about the good of every patient, and if he believes the duty of a pharmacist is to serve all pertinent needs of a patient, then he would certainly put aside any idea of excluding Mrs. Pinkham from his services. Regardless of the source of her medication, or her loyalties to him as a pharmacist, she has asked for assistance and Bill needs to deliver. Merely shunting Mrs. Pinkham back to the mail-order service would cause her discomfort and possibly harm from the lack of immediate information.

## Observing truthfulness in placebo therapy

Prescriptions for placebo drugs that have no overt pharmacological activity pose special problems for pharmacists, both with regard to the deception that is inherent in placebo therapy and the lack of truthfulness that attends such therapy. Pharmacist-historian Gregory J. Higby concludes that "placebos are generally harmful to the patient" and "physicians and pharmacists should discourage the use of placebic medication."[27] This sweeping indictment of placebo therapy is underscored by Veatch who argues that their use would become "almost morally impossible" if society were to allow no exceptions from the duty of truthfulness. Under these strict conditions, therefore, placebo therapy would be morally acceptable only in those cases where the patient has consented to be deceived.[28] Although pharmacists do not often encounter placebo prescriptions in their everyday practice, concerned pharmacists should be prepared to respond to these potentially sensitive drug orders in an appropriate and professional manner.

### Case 3.5: Interpreting Placebo Therapy

*"I hope this new drug takes effect quickly."*

Alex St. Martin is a 19-year-old exchange student who is in the hospital recovering from abdominal surgery for a gunshot wound. Alex is recovering nicely but is now experiencing "a great deal of pain" according to his continuing calls to the nursing station. Alex's surgeon, Dr. Beaumont, doesn't believe in using pain-killers in "these kinds of cases," since the pain is probably transient and will subside in a few days. Nevertheless, Dr. Beaumont promises Alex some suitable therapy and summons clinical pharmacist Hank Lincoln to the nursing station where he dictates the following order: "Prepare a 30 ml vial of Sterile Distilled Water . . . label it as Meperidine 50 mg/ml. . . Sig: 50 mg prn for pain . . . do not refill." As Hank hands the completed prescription to the primary care nurse Alex recognizes him and exclaims, "I hope this new drug takes effect quickly!" What is Hank's responsibility to Alex at this point? Should he reveal the nature of the medication to the primary care nurse? Should Hank have refused to prepare the placebo injection initially? If so, under what grounds?

**Commentary:** In a society where strict adherence to truthfulness is demanded of health-care professionals, the use of placebo therapy would be impossible. The 1994 Code of Ethics for Pharmacists, with its strong appeal to covenantal ethics and pharmaceutical care, expects pharmacists to respect patient autonomy, resist any tendency to be paternalistic, and certainly assume the role of patient advocate even to the point of refusing to participate in placebo therapy regimens. Therapeutic conflicts such as seen in this case will offer the most experienced pharmacist the opportunity to test personally held values with those of the larger medical community. Hank Lincoln is confronted with a situation that requires a nearly immediate response, voiding any real time for Hank to reflect or rely upon a critical analysis. Cases such as this one stress the need for all health professionals to identify their personal value system and how it affects their practice standards. Does Hank have time to discuss the situation with Alex, or is it enough for him to soothe Alex with something like, "Alex, Dr. Beaumont is one of the finest physicians in this hospital and this medication is one of the most effective he could have selected."

### Case 3.6: Identifying Placebo Therapy

*"This drug doesn't seem to be working for me."*

Fred Stearns, the chief pharmacist for National Drug Services, seemed to be nervous as he approached one of the patients standing in the counseling area of his large urban pharmacy. The patient waiting for him was Mr. Munyon, one of the nicest people that Fred has had the pleasure to serve. Unfortunately, Mr. Munyon had suffered a terrible accident, after which he had become extremely tense and prone to disturbing emotional outbursts that were controlled with large doses of a tranquilizer. Recently, Mr. Munyon's physician requested Fred to begin to replace portions of the tranquilizer with lactose, doing so in a manner that would preclude detection by Mr. Munyon. Fred developed an elegant approach, first replacing 10% of the active ingredients with inert lactose, then 20%, 30%, and 40%, until last week the prescription that he prepared was entirely composed of lactose. In order to maintain the appearance of continuing to supply the same drug, Fred continued to charge Mr. Munyon the same price for the medication, even though the cost of the inert ingredient was a fraction of cost of the original drug. As he approached Mr. Munyon he noticed that he looked uncomfortable and tense. Before he could even properly acknowledge Mr. Munyon's presence he heard, "Fred, this drug doesn't seem to working for me anymore. What's wrong?" Was Fred correct in complying with the physician's request to deceive Mr. Munyon? How should he answer the patient at this moment? Are there other alternatives that a pharmacist might pursue?

**Commentary:** Some cases of placebo therapy may carry with them additional difficulties that go beyond or add to the apparent deceiving of the patient. One such difficulty that may be encountered in pharmacy practice is outlined in this case where the cost of the drug supplied becomes part of the deceit plan. Even the experienced pharmacist who supports placebo therapy will often waffle when asked how to resolve this situation. Fred Stearns is faced with the distressing possibility of having to discuss with Mr. Munyon not only the deceit of the medication but also the intentional excessive pricing. Fred's initial response might be to quickly fall back on the prescribing physician, relying upon him to provide a full explanation and thus skirt the unpleasant prospect of confession. Like all ethical dilemmas, this case will require a careful consideration of the basic problem: Who is being harmed and by what action? Whose value system is being honored and whose is being ignored?

## Reconciling guilt feelings

As noted above, moral philosophers encourage health professionals to engage in not only obligatory ethical conduct, but also in acts that are morally optional, acts which would be meritorious and even praiseworthy. Pharmacists often encounter situations in which they must decide how much information they should provide the patient without seriously compromising either therapy or the duty of fidelity. The inevitable compromises often produce feelings of guilt or shame in the conscientious pharmacist, and may lead to feelings of professional inadequacy in the clinical setting.

### Case 3.7: Providing Comprehensive Drug Information

*"How dangerous could this prescription be?"*

Jon Swift, a 45-year-old paraplegic, was prescribed several months' supply of a tricyclic antidepressant to assist in coping with the divorce of his wife and the alienation of his teenaged son. While being counseled in the use of his drug, Jon asked the young pharmacist Jack Milhau a direct question: "How dangerous could this prescription be?" Jack carefully revealed that tricyclics may pose a problem of toxicity due to the fact that they are not easily removed from the body in cases of emergency. Soon after the discussion, Jon ingested a large amount of the drug and died, the result of an apparent suicide. Upon hearing of the incident, Jack felt guilty and somehow partially responsible. What duty did Jack have to inform Jon about his drug, knowing of his serious depression?

Commentary: This actual case, reported by a Montana pharmacist, demonstrates the serious situations pharmacists may encounter as they strive to provide the best possible care. There is little question that the Code of Ethics for Pharmacists expects pharmacists to promote the good of every patient in a caring and compassionate manner, and certainly to respect the right of self-determination. Providing factual information to patients about the drugs they are taking is no more than expected and fulfills many of these mandates. Yet this approach, as seen in this case, may lead to unanticipated difficulties. As a compassionate pharmacist, Jack Milhau could justify his behavior in this case by appealing to his personal value of veracity, declaring that Jon had the right to the information he had requested. Why is Jack troubled by the event? What is causing his feeling of "guilt" and is it justifiable, or is Jack feeling no more than remorse caused by the tragic pathway taken by Jon? Other possible responses to the request for detailed information might have had consequences that are just as horrific and much more difficult to defend. If Jack had decided to deflect the request in some way by referring Jon back to the prescribing physician or providing a "nonanswer," would this "square" Jack more clearly in his ethical responsibility?

### Case 3.8: Providing Incomplete Drug Information

*"The side effects associated with this drug are rare."*

In filling new prescriptions for oral contraceptives, pharmacist Ed Parrish is always particularly careful to inform his patients of not only how these drugs should be taken, but also their common side effects. Ann Besant, a high-school senior, presents Ed with such a prescription, but seems more apprehensive than other young patients Ed has counseled. As he concludes his usual advice and cautions about the drug, Ann inquires hesitantly, "Are there any other side effects I should know about?" Ed is aware that oral contraceptives may cause life-threatening embolisms in rare cases, but has some reason to believe that Ann might be hesitant to take her new medication if he reveals this information. "The side effects associated with this drug are rare," Ed replies after a short pause. Ann thanks him and pays for her prescription. Later, upon reflection, Ed feels somewhat ashamed that he dodged Ann's direct question. Why is Ed so troubled? Should he have provided Ann with complete information about the drugs untoward effects? If so, should Ed make an attempt to contact Ann?

**Commentary:** Patients' requests for specific information may be the most frequently encountered pharmacy practice situation that invite ethical dilemmas. In such situations, pharmacists have to "sift" through long lists of drug product data to produce a meaningful and effective exchange with the patient. The challenge of balancing the ethical "duty to inform" with the legal "duty to inform" is no doubt one of the most awesome in professional pharmacy practice. Ed Parrish's feeling of shame should signify to him a conflict, perhaps a compromise, with his personal standards. By reviewing the foundation upon which he based his decision-making he may be able to reconcile his feelings. Regardless, Ed must be able to defend his action with reasonable clarity and supportable facts.

## Maintaining patient confidentiality

Of all the values associated with pharmacy practice, patient confidentiality is the most easily identified and the most prevalent. Whether the duty to maintain patient confidentiality is absolute or can be abridged under certain special circumstances, remains an open question. In today's fractionated system of health care, pharmacists must be particularly alert to conflicts that may arise from compromised patient confidences.

### Case 3.9: Establishing the Boundaries of Confidentiality

*"What is my wife's prescription for, Doc?"*

Dick Cabot has just picked up his annual summary of medical expenditures from Zeke Sargent's pharmacy to assist him in preparing his tax returns. As he begins to leave, he stops, comes back, and points to one particular entry on the tax record printout. "What is my wife's prescription for, Doc?" Zeke looks at the entry, a prescription for a mild antibiotic. "I'm sorry, Dick," Zeke replied after a short pause, "I'm afraid I can't tell you that. Perhaps you should ask your wife." "Why won't you tell me?" Dick retorts with some warmth. "Aren't you supposed to be the expert on drugs?" Is Zeke correct in maintaining Mrs. Cabot's confidentiality, even to her husband? Under what conditions could Zeke release this information? If the drug were used in treating a vaginal infection or venereal disease would these conditions change?

Commentary: The keeping of confidences is one of the major aspects of fidelity, and certainly one of the classical ethical requirements of professional health-care ethics. The 1994 Code of Ethics for Pharmacists pledges "serving the patient in a private and confidential manner" and eliminates previous code exceptions of "except when it is in the interest of the patient." As such, the 1994 Code leaves pharmacists with the dilemma that no client-centered reasons are sufficient to permit breaking confidences. As pharmacists become more involved with principle- and virtue-based code statements, they will encounter other situations that may beg for exception, such as a case where breaking a confidence may benefit another individual or benefit society. Zeke Sargent is confronted with a simple case of whether Mrs. Cabot's husband has a right to information that may be protected by a confidence. Experienced pharmacists will ordinarily discuss the matter in a manner that would ultimately calm the inquirer and at the same time protect the confidence of the patient.

### Case 3.10: Restricting Access to Patient Information

*"Can I flip through your new scripts?"*

Over the past five years, Dick Stabler, owner of the S & L Pharmacy, has enjoyed the friendship of Jack Farr, a medical service representative for a large pharmaceutical firm. Dick and Jack are frequent golfing partners and have served together on committees of their local pharmaceutical association. Today, Jack drops in for a cup of coffee and mentions that he has been trying to introduce a new prescription specialty to area physicians without much success. Although his company provides him with sales figures on the new drug, he would like to identify prescribing patterns of the physicians in his area, and thus be able to target his marketing efforts. "Can I flip through your new scripts, Dick?" Jack asks casually. Dick wants to help his friend, but feels a little troubled. What should his response to Jack be? Under what circumstances, if any, should Dick open his prescription records to others?

**Commentary:** Compiling and safeguarding medical records often raises important and controversial issues such as who is the "moral" owner and what are the boundaries of disclosure. In the profession of pharmacy, the compilation and securing of prescription records is the keystone of practice. Not only the original information supplied by the physician but also notes by pharmacists may be added to any prescription record; with computerized systems, these prescription records have expanded into more elaborate and more informative medication profiles. Furthermore, aggressive marketing ploys from third-party agencies with requests for specific prescribing information have ostensibly intruded into the picture. Dick Stabler is now confronted with a situation that will certainly test his friendship with John and at the same time provide an opportunity for explaining his role as a patient advocate. He should be able to defend the confidentiality of patient records by resorting to basic moral principles or at least to the Code of Ethics for Pharmacists.

## Concluding Remarks

As we have seen, the pharmacist-patient relationship is both complex and potentially troublesome with regard to the moral and ethical issues that pharmacists face in their everyday practice. We have suggested that the moral basis for this relationship initially lay within traditional moral principles reflected in codes of professional conduct and ethics. Despite the conflicts engendered by recent shifts in their professional functions, contemporary pharmacists may feel more comfortable employing a virtue-based ethical system in which the rights of the patients are balanced by pharmacists' personal values, particularly as they can be applied to good patient care and emerging community needs.

## Study Questions

3.1 Would there be a different set of pharmacist duties toward the patient if the relationship was described as a pharmacist-*client* relationship?

3.2 Describe the moral basis for a pharmacist-patient relationship in your own words.

3.3 What guidelines, if any, should control your casual conversations with other health-care practitioners concerning patient prescription records? Are these conversations exempt from the general duty of confidentiality?

## Situations for Analysis

3.1 A young pharmacist accepts a position with a pharmacy that has a well-established reputation for knowing its patients. The pharmacy follows a policy of charging according to what the owner thinks the patient can afford to pay. Prices for nonbranded items are higher for those who can afford to pay, while the less well-to-do are charged prices close to cost.

3.2 A pharmacist agrees to serve as a consultant to a skilled nursing facility that has been operating for about ten years. In her initial review of the medication regimens, she notices that all patients receive an expensive, extemporaneously prepared skin lotion monthly. The pharmacist believes that the lotion is not only expensive, but worthless.

3.3 A pharmacist receives a prescription for a fertility drug from a Medicaid recipient with four young dependents. The pharmacist grudgingly fills the prescription, but counsels the patient on the advisability of submitting to a tubal ligation.

# References

1.  See, for example, "The Physician-Patient Relationship as a Narrative," Chapter 10 in Howard Brody, *Stories of Sickness* (New Haven and London: Yale University Press, 1987), pp. 171-81; Jay Katz, *The Silent World of Doctor and Patient* (New York: The Free Press, 1984); and Anne H. Bishop and John R. Scudder, Jr., eds., *Caring, Curing, Coping: Nurse, Physician, Patient Relationships* (University, Alabama: University of Alabama Press, 1985).
2.  See "The Professional and Patient Relationship," Chapter 7 in Tom L. Beauchamp and James F. Childress, *Principles of Biomedical Ethics*, 5th ed. (New York and Oxford: Oxford University Press, 2001), pp. 312.
3.  William F. May, *The Physician's Covenant: Images of the Healer in Medical Ethics* (Philadelphia: The Westminster Press, 1983), pp. 106-44, especially pp. 115-16.
4.  Brody notes that "having a rational plan of life is very much the same thing as . . . stating in advance the detailed obituary that one would like to have written . . . after death." See Brody, *Stories of Sickness* (n. 1), pp. 48-49.
5.  In three separate public opinion polls conducted between 1981 and 1985, respondents rated pharmacists second only to clergymen with regard to honesty and ethical standards. See I[rving] R[ubin], "Stat-o-Grams: 3-in-a-Row Gallup Polls of the Public on Honesty & Ethics: Pharmacists (Still No. 2) Edge Closer to Clergymen (No. 1)," *Pharmacy Times 51*:10 (October, 1985), p. 1. By 1990, the situation had improved, as pharmacists "received the highest rating out of 25 professions in the past four years." See "A Vote of Confidence: Pharmacists Shine in NACDS/Gallup Poll," *Pharmacy Update 1*:2 (July 30, 1990), p. 14. Some observers urged caution: "One might ask what we, as pharmacists, do to deserve such a standing in the public's collective eye." See J. Chris Bradbury, "The Latest Gallup Survey," *American Journal of Pharmaceutical Education 54*:2

(Summer, 1990), p. 217. Since 1999, pharmacists have placed second only to nurses, still commanding the respect of two-thirds of the American public. See Darren K. Carlson, "Nurses Remain at Top on Honesty and Ethics Poll," *Gallup Poll Monthly*, No. 422 (November, 2000), pp. 45-48.

6. May, *The Physician's Covenant* (n. 3), p. 116.

7. Mary Carolyn Cooper, "Covenantal Relationships: Grounding for the Nursing Ethic," *Advances in Nursing Science 10*:4 (July, 1988), pp. 48-49.

8. The concept of a broadly based information network for pharmacy was articulated by T. Donald Rucker in 1972, who stated that "no more powerful tool could be developed to aid qualified practitioners [to] cross the threshold from commercialism into the area of clinical pharmacy." T. Donald Rucker, "A Model Information System for Prescription Drug Services," *The Wisconsin Pharmacist 51*:12 (December, 1972), p. 412.

9. Jennifer Taylor Fix, "Nurturing the Patient/Pharmacist Relationship" [letter to the editor], *American Pharmacy NS29*:5 (May, 1989), p. 314. "[The] pressure for a large volume of prescription orders may inhibit the pharmacist's availability for customer service," Fix stresses.

10. Edward C. Elliott, *The General Report of the Pharmaceutical Survey, 1946-49* (Washington, D.C.: American Council on Education, 1950), p. 4.

11. Edmund D. Pellegrino and David C. Thomasma, *A Philosophical Basis of Medical Practice: Toward a Philosophy and Ethic of the Healing Professions* (New York and Oxford: Oxford University Press, 1981), p. 178.

12. Robert M. Veatch, "Ethical Principles in Pharmacy Practice," in *The Challenge of Ethics in Pharmacy Practice*, Publication No. 8, New Series, edited by Robert A. Buerki (Madison, Wisconsin: American Institute of the History of Pharmacy, 1985), pp. 18-19.

13. "APhA Code of Ethics," *Journal of the American Pharmaceutical Association NS9*:11 (November, 1969), p. 552. Also see [Forrest T. Patterson], "In Summary . . . Workshop Discussions," *Journal of the American Pharmaceutical Association NS8*:3 (March, 1968), pp. 142-44.

14. Frankena expands the concept of beneficence to include four distinct levels of good acts: 1) the duty to not inflict evil or harm, 2) the duty to prevent evil or harm, 3) the duty to remove evil, and 4) the duty to do or promote good. William K. Frankena, *Ethics*, 2nd ed. (Englewood Cliffs, New Jersey: Prentice-Hall, Inc., 1973), p. 47.

15. Edward Parrish, "Ethical Analysis," *Proceedings of the American Pharmaceutical Association 6* (1857), p. 149. Parrish's analysis may be the first serious consideration of American pharmacists' moral responsibilities.

16. For a detailed discussion of the concept of justice, see "The Principle of Justice," Chapter 6 in Beauchamp and Childress, *Principles of Biomedical Ethics* (n. 2), pp. 225-82.

17. Parrish, "Ethical Analysis" (n. 15), p. 149. Parrish considered such pharmacists as participating in "the moral obloquy which among enlightened and conscientious people attaches to the charlatan and quack."

18. Seymour Banner and Carol Levine, "Pharmacy, Science & Society: Medicaid 'Boycotts': Economics and Ethics in Conflict," *U.S. Pharmacist 4*:3 (March, 1979), p. 71.

19. Beauchamp and Childress, *Principles of Biomedical Ethics* (n. 2), pp. 79-80.

20. Veatch, "Ethical Principles in Pharmacy Practice" (n. 12), p. 16.
21. "Code of Ethics of the American Pharmaceutical Association," *Journal of the American Pharmaceutical Association 11*:9 (September, 1922), p. 728; and [1969] "APhA Code of Ethics" (n. 13), p. 552.
22. Robert M. Veatch, "Pharmacy Ethics: Maintaining Patient Confidentiality in a Case of Potential Substance Abuse: Analysis and Commentary," *American Journal of Hospital Pharmacy 46*:1 (January, 1989), pp. 118-19. Also see American Medical Association, "5.05: Confidentiality," *Current Opinions of the Judicial Council of the American Medical Association* (Chicago: American Medical Association, 1989), p. 19.
23. Section II, "Code of Ethics for Pharmacists," approved October 27, 1994 by the membership of the American Pharmaceutical Association.
24. Daniel Callahan, "Ethics and Health Care: The Next Twenty Years," in *Pharmacy in the 21st Century: Planning for an Uncertain Future*, edited by Clement Bezold, Jerome A. Halperin, Howard L. Binkley, and Richard A. Ashbaugh (Bethesda, Maryland: Institute for Alternative Futures and Project HOPE, 1985), p. 83.
25. Edmund D. Pellegrino and David C. Thomasma, *For the Patient's Good: The Restoration of Beneficence in Health Care* (New York and Oxford: Oxford University Press, 1988), p. 112. Without agreeing on the nature of the good, the authors add, society "can hardly know what a 'disposition' to do the right and good may mean." *Ibid.*
26. Robert G. Mrtek, "The American Institute of the History of Pharmacy and Its Role in Ethics," *American Journal of Pharmaceutical Education 53*:1 (Spring, 1989), p. 70.
27. Gregory J. Higby, "Placebo Prescriptions and the Problems They Present to Community Pharmacists," *Journal of Social and Administrative Pharmacy 3*:1 (1985), p. 30. "When shown how placebo therapy can harm the patient, society at large, and the medical profession, physicians may begin setting aside this and other deceptive practices." *Ibid.*, p. 39.
28. Robert M. Veatch, *A Theory of Medical Ethics* (New York: Basic Books, Inc., 1981), pp. 220-21.

# Suggested Readings

Childress, James F. "The Place of Autonomy in Bioethics." *Hastings Center Report 20*:1 (January-February, 1990), pp. 12-17.

Foster, Thomas S., and Raehl, Cynthia L. "Legal and Ethical Issues in Clinical Pharmacy Research: Informed Consent, Part I." *Drug Intelligence and Clinical Pharmacy 14*:1 (January, 1980), pp. 40-43; Part II, *ibid.*, *14*:2 (February, 1980), pp. 122-25.

Haddad, Amy Marie. "Case Study: Keeping Confidences." *American Pharmacy NS33*:12 (December, 1993), pp. 50-52.

Higby, Gregory J. "Placebo Prescriptions and the Problems They Present to Community Pharmacists." *Journal of Social and Administrative Pharmacy 3*:1 (1985), pp. 30-40.

Manolakis, Michael L., McCart, Gary M., and Veatch, Robert M. "Pharmacy Ethics: Pharmacist's Refusal to Serve Patient with AIDS." *American Journal of Hospital Pharmacy 47*:1 (January, 1990), pp. 151-54.

McCart, Gary M., Clyne, Kurt E., and Veatch, Robert M. "Pharmacy Ethics: Maintaining Patient Confidentiality in a Case of Potential Substance Abuse." *American Journal of Hospital Pharmacy 46*:1 (January, 1989), pp. 116-19.

Resnik, David B., Resnik, Susan P., Arnold, Robert, Nissen, Julia, and Haupt, Bridget. "Case Studies: What's a Pharmacist to Do?" *Hastings Center Report 19*:3 (May-June, 1989), pp. 38-40.

Veatch, Robert M. *The Foundations of Justice: Why the Retarded and the Rest of Us Have Claims to Equality.* New York and Oxford: Oxford University Press, 1986.

Veatch, Robert M. "Pharmacy, Science & Society: Informed Consent: The Emerging Principles." *U.S. Pharmacist 6*:3 (March, 1981), pp. 78-80.

Veatch, Robert M., and Haddad, Amy [M.]. *Case Studies in Pharmacy Ethics.* New York: Oxford University Press, 1999.

Wertheimer, A[lbert] I., and Seradell, J[oaquima]. "Commentary: Prescribed Drugs and Patient Consent," *Journal of Clinical Pharmacy and Therapeutics 13*:1 (1988), pp. 1-4.

# CHAPTER 4

# ETHICAL CONSIDERATIONS IN PROFESSIONAL COMMUNICATION

As suggested in earlier chapters, it is clear from the historical record that American pharmacists saw themselves as more than mere shopkeepers. From the earliest years of the Republic, pharmacists set high self-imposed standards regarding the nature of the health-care information they supplied to their customers. In 1824, for example, the founders of the Philadelphia College of Pharmacy became concerned about the "extravagant pretensions and false assertions" of the wildly variant versions of the popular English patent medicines that had become a mainstay of American self-medication. To correct such abuses, the College published a booklet of standardized formulas for several of these nostrums, including "suitable papers of directions" for their patrons' use.[1] In so doing, the College not only demonstrated a concern for truth in advertising, but may have originated the concept of the patient package insert. In 1857, Edward Parrish asked if it was "morally right" for a pharmacist who has the "confidence of the poor and ignorant in his neighborhood" to sell "costly and often worse than useless medicines" which are "plausibly and insidiously recommended" by the public press.[2] The 1874 edition of Parrish's *A Treatise on Pharmacy*, noting that the public generally had "little opportunity" to acquaint themselves with drugs that were "for so many centuries wrapped in obscure nomenclature," encouraged the pharmacist to "interest inquiring minds in the commercial, botanical, and chemical history of the articles he dispenses, and to explain their uses."[3]

This thread of concern for truth-telling and communicating complete, objective drug information to the public ran through the fabric of American pharmacy practice during the nineteenth century. As medical and pharmaceutical practices became defined by state law, however, a new—albeit cautious—symbiotic relationship began to develop between physicians and pharmacists, particularly with regard to the scope of their respective practices. Physicians

101

were expected to diagnose and prescribe; pharmacists were expected to compound and dispense. Those who ventured out of their
domain were denounced as "physician dispensers" and "counter-
prescribers."[4] This rigid separation of professional functions had an
unanticipated negative impact upon the relationship between pharmacists and their patients, particularly with regard to the nature
of their professional communications.

## Communication as an ethical standard

Paradoxically, for over 150 years, American pharmacists appeared
to hold a double standard with regard to the nature of their professional communications with the public. On one hand, pharmacists
forswore secret remedies and denounced other evils of the patent
medicine trade through their codes of ethics and other public statements. On the other hand, these same codes threw a shroud of secrecy over the pharmacist-patient relationship with regard to discussing the nature of their patrons' prescribed medicines.
Overshadowing both these standards of practice was a set of rigid
ethical rules that outlined a code of professional discretion, particularly with regard to errors in practice.

**Professional discretion as an ideal.** The early codes of ethics of
the Philadelphia College of Pharmacy (1848) and the American
Pharmaceutical Association (1852) set the groundwork for pharmaceutical standards of practice, some of which were later set
down in law. Pharmacists and physicians were supposed to look after each others' interests, particularly with regard to errors in practice. The Philadelphia code enjoined apothecaries to correct physicians' errors "without the knowledge of the patient, so that the
physician may be screened from censure." Physicians, too, were
told they had a duty to "stand between the apothecary and the patient" in screening pharmacists' errors. More pointedly, the Association code stated that "the apothecary should always, when he
deems an error has been made, consult the physician before proceeding," adding that the pharmacist had a duty to "accomplish
the interview without compromising the reputation of the physician." Physicians, likewise, when discovering pharmacists' errors,
"should feel bound to screen them from undue censure, unless the
result of culpable negligence."[5]
   While both early codes discountenanced the use of "secret formulae" and "practices arising from a quackish spirit," the practice
of maintaining an aura of secrecy in patient communications ran

much deeper. The Western tradition of *privileged communication* between patient and practitioner, an artifact of the ancient priestly role of the physician, is based upon the conviction that knowledge of a person's private life gained in the course of professional services belongs to the person served. This trust is often curiously perverted by some physicians who express righteous indignation at any attempt to pry patient information from them while denying this same information to its rightful owner, the patient.

Physicians also felt it was "not seemly" to discuss their treatment plans with their patients, a conviction reflected in their Latinized prescriptions. The use of Latin in prescription writing was usually defended on three grounds: First, Latin was touted as the international "language of science," allowing pharmacists to compound the prescriptions of physicians of any nationality. Second, the Latin names of medicines were seen as fixed and not subject to change. Finally, and perhaps most telling, the use of Latin in prescriptions afforded secrecy. "This last reason should be remembered and respected by the pharmacist," the redoubtable Wilbur L. Scoville wrote in the 1914 edition of his text, *The Art of Compounding.* "Inquiries regarding the composition of and nature of a prescription should be answered with caution," Scoville continued. "It may be objectionable to answer frankly such questions when asked by people of high intelligence and with honorable motives but in most cases an evasive reply, which conveys little or no information, is advisable."[6] This and similar advice persisted in pharmacy textbooks well into the 1950s.

The standard of nondisclosure of prescription information was first embodied in the 1922 Code of Ethics of the American Pharmaceutical Association, affecting generations of practitioners. "Never discuss the therapeutic effect of a Physician's prescription with a patron nor disclose details of composition which the Physician has withheld," the Code stated frankly. Pharmacists were expected to refer patients and their questions back to their physicians. Thirty years later, this standard had not changed: The 1952 Association Code declared that the ethical pharmacist "does not discuss the therapeutic effects or composition of a prescription with a patient. When such questions are asked, he suggests that the qualified practitioner is the proper person with whom such matters should be discussed."[7]

Once the concept of therapeutic secrecy had been incorporated into the pharmacy code of ethics, many practitioners and well-meaning pharmacy educators alike began devising novel approaches to deal with inquisitive patients, approaches that were often also intended to raise the stature of pharmacists in the eyes of the public. In the 1937 edition of their textbook, *Principles of Pharmacy*, for example, Henry V. Arny and Robert P. Fischelis provided advice to pharmacy students in the form of a "case study":

A man who once had a prescription wrongly compounded insisted on sitting behind the prescription counter watching the compounder, so as to keep tab. To make things still safer, he usually plied the compounder with questions. The new clerk was a young man just from college; the man, more suspicious than ever, was more persistent in questioning. "What's this medicine?" he inquired, pointing to the then little-known abbreviation "antipy." "Oh," said the youth, nonchalantly, "that's Latin for the new medicine, phenyl-dim-ethyl-pyrazolon." From that day forth the man considered the youth the smartest and most reliable druggist in town.[8]

Resourceful practitioners and educators soon developed strategies for providing "noninformation" to patient inquiries. "The physician is really the one to whom the customer should address such questions," William J. Husa's *Pharmaceutical Dispensing* cautioned pharmacy students in 1951. "Since a direct refusal to answer such inquiries may offend or embarrass the customer, some pharmacists prefer to give a cheery but evasive reply which does not convey any unwarranted information."[9] Some schools of pharmacy in the 1950s even taught their students to parrot certain phrases designed to enhance the pharmacists' image while maintaining both professional discretion and the tacit support of the prescribing physician.[10]

**Forging new ethical standards.** By the 1960s, honest and forthright communication between pharmacists and patients began to emerge as a new practice standard. Various forces, some societal, some professional, continually nudged the minds and consciences of pharmacists, educators, and patients alike toward a new level of professional responsibility in pharmacy practice. The consumerism movement of the late 1960s, which demanded full disclosure of product and service information, the increasing sophistication of the public with regard to the drugs they were consuming, and the pharmacological revolution, particularly the introduction of psychoactive drugs and oral contraceptives, set the stage for a new, patient-centered practice of pharmacy. "Secrecy surrounding medicines, which was a part of earlier therapy, has almost disappeared," declared the 1966 text *Clinical Pharmacy: A Text for Dispensing Pharmacy.* "There is a growing tendency for the patient to know what specific medicine he is taking, and in a good number of circumstances, for the physician to tell him."[11] Despite this new ten-

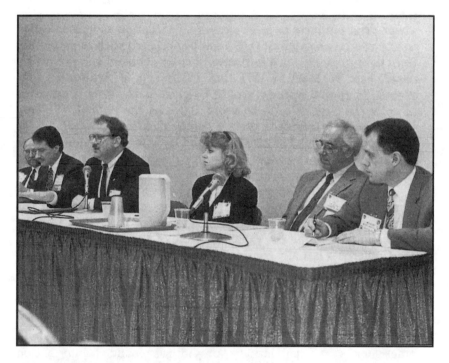

The Code of Ethics Review Committee held open hearings on the proposed Code of Ethics for Pharmacists as part of the 140th Annual Meeting and Exposition of the American Pharmaceutical Association in Dallas, Texas, 23 March 1993. Members included (left to right) William A. Zellmer, Calvin H. Knowlton, Joseph L. Fink, III (Chair), Elizabeth K. Keyes, Louis D. Vottero, and Michael L. Manolakis. Committee members not pictured are Beverly Mendoza, David G. Miller, and Jesse C. Vivian. (*Photograph courtesy of American Pharmaceutical Association.*)

dency toward openness, however, the old prohibitions still held sway. "The pharmacist should never indulge in criticisms or suggestions regarding the therapeutic action of a remedy or its value," the textbook continued, noting that "this lies outside the scope of pharmacy and undoubtedly will antagonize the physician."[12] Rather than encouraging pharmacists to discuss the therapeutic actions of drugs with their patients, however, the first editions of clinically oriented textbooks encouraged pharmacists to draw upon their scientific knowledge in order to convey technical information about drug products to their patients. "Attention should be called to any special precautions that must be observed such as protection from light or storage in a refrigerator, color changes, and expiration date," Eric W. Martin's 1971 text *Dispensing of Medication* suggested. "A special warning should be given if the drug is expected to color the feces or urine to avoid alarming the patient."[13] These well-meaning attempts at patient communication, however, fell far short of the public's increasing demand for information about their medications. Complete openness with patients would wait upon the development of a new ethical standard for pharmacy practice.

A special Conference on Ethics convened by the American Pharmaceutical Association in 1967 focussed attention upon the perceived inadequacies of the 1952 revision of the APhA Code of Ethics in monitoring the expanding role of the pharmacist. While the Conference initially considered merely updating the Code to reflect emerging ethical issues, the participants soon shifted their attention to drafting an entirely new code. The now troublesome prohibition on discussion of therapeutic effect and composition of prescribed drugs with patients was "critically attacked." Participants recommended that pharmacists be allowed to assist both practitioners and patients by providing expanded information about drugs. The "inflexible prohibition" on informing patients about their prescriptions was modified to allow pharmacists "to use professional judgment in deciding whether to discuss medication with the patient." Moreover, participants recommended that "the pharmacist willingly make available his expert knowledge of medication to his patrons and health professionals."[14] The new Code, drafted by the Association's Judicial Board and presented to its House of Delegates in 1968, dropped the now controversial language prohibiting pharmacists from discussing "therapeutic effects or composition of a prescription" with their patients. In its place, the new Code expanded an earlier concept of utilizing professional knowledge:

A pharmacist should always strive to perfect and enlarge his professional knowledge. He should utilize and make available this knowledge as may be required in accordance with his best professional judgment.

While silent upon the specific issue of patient counseling, the Judicial Board clearly recognized that "the pharmacist has a duty to employ this knowledge at times when it is required." Moreover, the Board expected the pharmacist to "make his professional knowledge available to patients in circumstances where it is in the best interest of the patient, as determined according to the professional judgment of the pharmacist."[15] While still retaining some paternalistic flavor, the new Code was ratified by the membership the following year, opening a new and exciting professional challenge to America's pharmacists.[16]

In August of 1989, the Joint Commission of Pharmacy Practitioners, representing a wide range of pharmacy practice organizations, expressed concerns about the 1969 APhA Code, a document it felt was no longer relevant as a guide to modern pharmacy practice. The Commission recommended the development of a "profession-wide code of ethics" for pharmacists which all professional associations could adopt.[17] The Commission also recommended that the American Pharmaceutical Association take the lead in developing the new code. The Association subsequently established a broad-based Code of Ethics Review Committee, including a wide range of pharmacy practitioners, pharmacist-lawyers, and state and national pharmaceutical association executives. The Committee adopted a deliberative process, seeking input from individual pharmacists, pharmacy educators, and national and state pharmaceutical associations. Successive drafts of a new "Code of Ethics for Pharmacists" were sent out for review and comment and presented at an open hearing at the March, 1993 Annual Meeting of the Association. A final draft of the new Code was approved by the Association's Board of Trustees in September, 1993 and approved by the membership in 1994.[18] While the 1969 Code was silent upon the issue of patient counseling, the new Code "recognizes the right of self-determination and individual self-worth" among patients, encouraging them to participate in decisions about their health. Moreover, the new Code encourages patient counseling, stressing that "a pharmacist communicates with patients in terms that are understandable."[19]

**The patient rights movement.** By the mid-1970s, a number of forces had converged that encouraged pharmacists to more fully share their professional knowledge with their patients. In 1973, the American Hospital Association's statement on a "Patient's Bill of Rights" proclaimed that patients have the right to obtain complete and current information concerning their diagnosis, treatment, and prognosis in terms they can be "reasonably expected to understand."[20] This statement bolstered the so-called "right to know" movement, stimulating more meaningful communication between patients and their health-care providers. Perfunctory, paternalistic monologues to secure patients' conformance with foreordained treatment plans would no longer be tolerated. "What is on the horizon is nothing less than a new theory of lay-professional relations," ethicist Robert M. Veatch exclaimed in 1979. "The new ethic for health professionals summarized in the patients' rights movement is no longer simply the protection of the patient from harm, but the preservation of autonomy and rights."[21]

Patients long accustomed to passively accepting perfunctory advice about their medications from their pharmacists were now encouraged to participate more fully in the decisions regarding their health care. Hospital pharmacists struggled trying to balance their traditional ethic of care and service with the new ethic of patients' rights. "The pharmacist must insure that all patients receive adequate information about the drugs they receive," the American Society of Hospital Pharmacists declared in its seminal "Minimum Standards for Pharmacies in Institutions," issued in 1977.[22] Two years later, the "Standards of Practice for the Profession of Pharmacy," issued jointly by the American Pharmaceutical Association and the American Association of Colleges of Pharmacy, delineated eighteen specific responsibilities regarding the "patient care functions" a pharmacist should perform to fulfill "the basic responsibilities of the profession."[23] While both documents outlined in great detail the responsibilities of pharmacists in the emerging patient-oriented practice of the late 1970s, they were silent on practice standards relating to the pharmacist's respect for patient autonomy.

The patient rights movement also manifested itself in lay participation in community health planning, lay appointments to state medical and pharmacy licensing boards, and the emergence of hospital ombudsmen to reconcile patient concerns. Within the arena of pharmacy practice, however, the patient rights movement generally focussed upon the rather narrow issues of prescription drug advertising, prescription price-posting, and the advertising of these prices through newspapers and other media. At the same time, pressed by dwindling profit margins and increased competition, chain and community pharmacists alike quietly eliminated the services traditionally associated with the practice of pharmacy, such as prescription delivery, personal charge accounts, 24-hour emergency service, and postal substations. By focussing upon the economic issues of their professional practice, they shifted the public's attention from traditional pharmacy services to the prices charged for prescription drugs and other medications. In retrospect, American pharmacists appear to have badly misinterpreted the underlying message of the patient rights movement: by treating prescription drugs as commodities the drugs became commodities in fact, undermining both the patient rights movement and the emerging ethical responsibilities associated with patient autonomy. Moreover, by creating such a strong commodity-based public image, pharmacists put into place a paradox that continues to haunt professional pharmacy practice today. As the drive toward healthcare reform continues, pharmacy leaders struggle to shift from this mercantile image of pharmacy practice to an image of a service-dominated practice that promotes improved patient outcomes.

## Communication as a practice standard

Communication between patients and their pharmacists has been a significant feature of American pharmacy practice for well over a century. As we have seen, the nature of this communication has shifted from a practice standard of professional secrecy or subtle obfuscation to a societal demand for full disclosure of drug and patient treatment information. Spurred on by the consumerism and patient rights movements, practicing pharmacists, pharmacy educators, and ethicists alike in the early 1970s became concerned with providing access to complete and accurate patient care information.

In a 1972 panel discussion entitled "Consumerism vs. Professionalism," for example, ethicist Thomas F. McMahon declared that the pharmacist was "changing priorities from the traditional role to an informational role." Noting that consumers also seemed to be seeking more information from their pharmacists, McMahon concluded that "the amount and kind of information dispersed and sought reveals a shift in the power centers between pharmacist and consumer. . . . Pharmacists willingly share their knowledge power with physicians and clients."[24] Three years later, the Report of the Study Commission on Pharmacy, *Pharmacists for the Future*, literally redefined the profession of pharmacy as a *"knowledge system* which renders a *health service*." The "pharmacist of the future" the Commission envisioned would be responsible for more than the delivery of a product to the ultimate consumer:

It is certain that he will be responsible for reinforcing the physician's instructions about drug therapies. . . . This will necessitate that he elicit information from the patient concerning his total use of drugs . . . . A more personal and continuing relationship with the patient should develop. The pharmacist will dispense drugs, and he will both dispense and elicit information concerning drugs usage and concerning the patient.[25]

The following year, the American Society of Hospital Pharmacists issued its comprehensive "Statement of Pharmacist-Conducted Patient Counseling," which argued that pharmacists have "a responsibility to properly inform patients about their drug therapy. . . . In addition, pharmacists must counsel patients in the proper selection of nonprescription drugs."[26]

Moreover, community and hospital pharmacists alike began to be concerned about the problem of noncompliance, an issue Dorothy L. Smith characterized in 1976 as "one of the major unsolved therapeutic problems facing medicine and pharmacy today."[27] Despite a spate of inconclusive research seeking to elicit the characteristics that might distinguish compliant patients from their noncompliant counterparts,[28] patient knowledge became identified as a necessary condition for compliance, but not always sufficient to ensure appropriate behavior.[29] By the 1980s, however, patient communication began to emerge as the quintessential ingredient in the pharmacist-patient relationship. Pharmacy faculty saw this emerging practice criterion as an opportunity to introduce course offerings in communications as they sought to graduate pharmacists with enhanced interpersonal communications skills.[30]

As an initial response to the internal and external demands for expanded drug information, many pharmacists made prescription drug package inserts or copies of the *Physicians' Desk Reference* available to their patients. Later, bombarded by queries about the rare side effects and exotic contraindications contained in these materials, pharmacists soon learned that mere *access* to drug information was an insufficient response to demands for expanded patient-care information. Subsequently, pharmacists became equally concerned about the *nature* and *extent* of the information they disclosed to their patients, and took pains to develop more appropriate patient education materials.

Once America's pharmacists became determined to share their drug expertise with their patients, they faced a number of

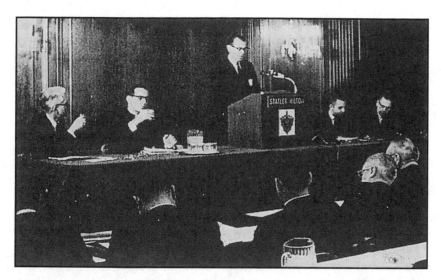

APhA President George W. Grider provides opening remarks at the APhA Conference on Ethics held in New York City, 29 November 1967. Other participants included (left to right) Bernard Barber, the Reverend Thomas F. McMahon, Robert F. Steeves, and George B. Griffenhagen. (*Photograph courtesy of American Pharmaceutical Association.*)

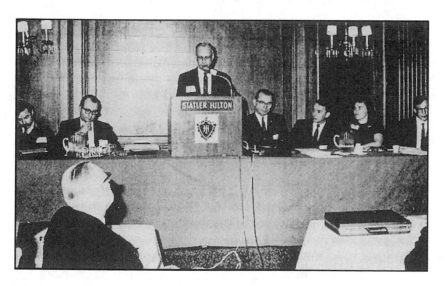

At the concluding session of the 1967 Conference on Ethics, Lloyd M. Parks, Chairman of the APhA Board of Trustees, asked the rhetorical question, "Where do we go from here?" (*Photograph courtesy of the American Pharmaceutical Association.*)

challenges associated with expanding their communication with patients. Some pharmacists encountered problems because of corporate restraints discouraging extended patient contact. Others faced formidable physical barriers such as high prescription counters or bullet-proof glass enclosures that made communication with patients difficult if not impossible. Still others felt inadequate because they lacked sufficient interpersonal communication skills. At about the same time, unfettered by codified ethical constraints, American pharmacists began experimenting with techniques of *patient counseling*, a patient-oriented activity that would later emerge as a new practice standard. This standard of patient counseling carried with it the distinct possibility of increased accountability for professional negligence, reflected by an expanded potential for professional malpractice suits and higher professional liability insurance premiums. Later, stimulated by an increasing awareness of patient autonomy and self-determination, pharmacists began placing a higher premium on the *outcomes* of counseling and the effects it might have on compliance with a drug regimen or other treatment plan, stressing the importance of information disclosure as a counseling element. As we will see, the *professional disclosure standard* for pharmacy practice draws its authority not only from legal and professional sources, but also from the realm of ethics.

**Legal duty to communicate.** In 1970, physician-lawyer Paul J. Matte, Jr., noted a "discernible and distinct trend" toward imposing a responsibility upon pharmacists for "protecting patients from error." Matte predicted that pharmacists would soon incur a legal duty to warn their patients of potential hazards, not unlike the doctrine of informed consent.[31] During the ensuing three decades, American courts have issued a persistent, yet confusing, series of rulings in cases concerning pharmacists' duty to warn in their communications with patients. Patients who sustained injuries from medications made claims against pharmacists because they did not properly communicate the hazards associated with the medications they dispensed. In 1991, Food and Drug Administration Commissioner David A. Kessler noted the increased expectation for patient counseling reflected in professional association practice standards. Pointing to a 1986 state supreme court ruling that pharmacists have a duty to inform patients about the risks of prescribed drugs, Kessler frankly stated that the primary responsibility for the proper use of drugs belongs to physicians and pharmacists.[32] In 1992, pharmacist-lawyer Brenda Raffath concluded that while pharmacists currently have no duty to warn under the liability

theories of negligence, strict liability, or implied warranty of fit-
ness, this immunity may be short-lived. Raffath noted that consumers of the 1990s began to assert their right to know the benefits
and risks associated with the use of a prescription drug.[33] Thus,
while some courts have held that pharmacists have an explicit duty
to warn of untoward effects caused by dispensed prescription medications, others hold that pharmacists are accountable for communicating or counseling their patients only about specific facts concerning the nature and use of these medications.[34] In their attempt
to adjudicate such questions, the courts generally apply one of two
standards for information disclosure to the practice of patient
counseling, the *professional practice standard* or the *reasonable person standard*. A third emerging standard, the *subjective disclosure
standard*, is based upon a body of thoughtful legal commentary
rather than case law.

The *professional practice standard* is established on the
premise that the traditional practices of a community of professionals will ultimately develop the needed standard of practice. In
this case, practicing pharmacists acting in the best interest of their
patients determine the appropriate information disclosure standard. This somewhat paternalistic approach depends upon the application of medical care standards rather than the application of
patients' rights. Ethicists Tom Beauchamp and James Childress
conclude that the custom in a profession establishes the amount
and kinds of information to be disclosed when applying the professional practice standard.[35] Some problems exist in applying this
standard, however. First, despite the efforts of professional associations, no generally accepted customary standard of information
disclosure exists for the extremely diverse range of practices represented within the profession of pharmacy. Moreover, as Beauchamp
and Childress point out, a custom-based practice standard could
perpetuate "pervasive negligence" within a profession, creating a
situation where a majority of well-meaning pharmacists could offer
a similar, yet inferior level of information.[36] As a legal standard,
therefore, the custom-based practice standard has the potential to
subvert the patient's right to adequate information, thus undermining or denying the patient's right to self-determination. In addition, the conceptual basis for a custom-based practice standard
in pharmacy is predicated on the sanguine belief that pharmacists
have the expertise to decide in all cases what sort of information
the patient actually wants to have. Consider, for example, a patient
who presents a prescription for methotrexate and then asks, "What
is this drug used for?" How do pharmacists determine the custom-

based practice standard that should be applied in this particular situation? Does the standard develop internally only after years of experience or is it based upon an informal system of shared values? Should the pharmacist respond to the patient's question directly or be evasive? Should the pharmacist refer such patients to their physicians or attempt to gather more information before replying?

A related problem associated with applying the custom-based practice standard lies with the source of the professional values that pharmacists exhibit in determining the nature and extent of information they divulge to patients. From what source do most practicing pharmacists draw the insights that contribute to their professional value systems? Experience suggests that novice pharmacists or interns will often fashion their responses after the example of their preceptors or other more experienced pharmacists who may serve as authority or role models. As a result, the custom-based standard becomes merely a restatement of another pharmacist's personal commitment to professional practice, a learned value. Both these problems seriously undermine the credibility of the professional practice standard as a legal basis for information disclosure in patient counseling.

The *reasonable person standard* relies upon a consideration of the kind and amount of information reasonable patients would want to know about the risks, alternatives, and consequences associated with taking their prescribed drugs. In contrast to the professional practice standard, the reasonable person standard shifts the determination of extent of information disclosure from the healthcare professional to the patient. In practice, this means that the pharmacist must divulge the kind of material information patients need in order to determine whether or not they will comply with a prescribed drug regimen. This standard permits patients to be the agents of their own decision-making in medical matters, thereby both respecting their autonomy and protecting their right to self-determination.[37]

While the reasonable person standard seems attractive from a patient rights perspective, certain problems plague its implementation. First, although the legal concept dates back to the eighteenth century, there is no generally accepted definition of what constitutes a "reasonable person" in a medical context. Second, physicians and pharmacists often find difficulty in discerning what a "reasonable person" would need to know to make good decisions regarding his or her health care. Finally, to what extent should physicians or pharmacists personalize their counseling to accommodate the specific needs of an individual patient, a patient who might not meet the polite legal fiction of the "reasonable person?" Many critics within the medical community have maintained that the reasonable person standard is not in the best interests of either patients or physicians and may be impossible to satisfy. Others raise questions about the standard and its ability to precisely define the duty of a health-care professional.[38]

In applying the reasonable person standard to the methotrexate case referred to above, for example, would the pharmacist counsel the patient differently if he or she knew that the patient was also undergoing treatment for severe depression? Can pharmacists be held accountable for constructing a reasonable person standard for each of their professional encounters in face of the myriad of individual characteristics their patients may display? Health-care professionals often have difficulty applying the abstract reasonable person standard to specific cases in their professional practice because they tend to personalize their professional encounters. As these practitioners tailor the standard to reflect the unique needs of each individual patient, they move away from the reasonable person standard and toward a more subjective standard for information disclosure.

The *subjective disclosure standard* requires health professionals to disclose whatever information is material to the counseling of a particular patient. Proponents of the subjective standard maintain that the patient's right to make decisions for personal reasons is not adequately protected by any other disclosure standard. Ethicists Ruth Fadden and Tom Beauchamp argue that if patients have a right to make individual, personal, or even unorthodox choices concerning their health care, they may need access to information that would not be considered relevant to either the professional practice standard or the reasonable person standard.[39] If our long-suffering patient requesting information about methotrexate had a history of noncompliant behavior, the pharmacist might choose to disclose more information about the dangers of irregular methotrexate therapy. Under the subjective disclosure standard, health-care professionals are obliged to disclose information a particular patient desires or needs to know, so long as there is a reasonable connection between these desires and needs for information and what the health-care professional should know about the patient's position. The moral question is not whether the information necessarily would have led the patient to forego therapy, but rather whether the information was necessary for this patient's informed decision, regardless of outcome. Despite the many problems that plague the subjective disclosure standard in law, Beauchamp and Childress find it "a preferable moral standard of disclosure" that supports the principle of respect for autonomy, because it "acknowledges the independent informational needs and desires of persons in the process of making difficult decisions."[40]

The subjective disclosure standard is reflected in two sections of the 1990 Omnibus Budget Reconciliation Act (OBRA), items of federal legislation that promise to redefine or even transform traditional medical and pharmaceutical practices in the United States. Section 4206, the so-called "Patient Self-Determination Act of 1990," requires hospitals, health maintenance organizations, community clinics, and other health-care providers to furnish written information to their Medicare patients regarding their right to accept or refuse medical or surgical treatment and their right to formulate "advance medical directives," instructions explaining how they wish to be treated if they become too ill to express their wishes.[41] In short, the Act formalizes the process by which health-care institutions provide information to their patients, institutionalizing a standard of disclosure which has as its goal an honest and deeply-held respect for patient self-determination. This dramatic shift in the health-care standard for information disclosure may revolutionize the relationship between health-care providers and their patients, redefining the institutional commitment to patient autonomy beyond mere conformity to minimal informed consent requirements.

Section 4401 of OBRA requires participating states to establish drug utilization review systems, including counseling standards under which pharmacists must offer to discuss certain matters with their Medicaid patients or their caregivers; many of these enhanced practice standards have been extended to the general public by changes in state pharmacy practice acts or state board regulations. Specifically, the Act requires pharmacists to perform a "prospective drug utilization review" for these patients, encompassing the complete range of their intended drug therapy, including any over-the-counter medications they may be taking. Pharmacists must complete these reviews prior to dispensing new drugs. Moreover, the Act requires pharmacists to exercise their professional judgment by asking them to decide what information is significant to the intended drug therapy of these patients. Although the legislation provides pharmacists with the foundation upon which they may develop a standard for subjective disclosure based on professional judgment, it also mandates certain specific "significant matters" which must be disclosed. These items include not only a complete description of the medication, its dosage, route of administration, and the duration of therapy, but also any special directions and precautions for preparation, administration, and use by the patient. In addition, pharmacists must explain common severe adverse effects, interactions, or therapeutic contraindications patients may encounter, including advice as to how these adverse effects may be avoided, and the action required if they occur. Moreover, pharmacists must explain techniques for self-monitoring drug therapy, including the proper action to be taken in the event of a missed dose. Pharmacists must also make a "reasonable effort" to obtain, record, and maintain at least the name, address, telephone number, date of birth (or age), and gender of these patients, their individual medical history, where significant, including disease state or states, known allergies and drug reactions, and a comprehensive list of their medications and relevant medical devices. Finally, pharmacists are supposed to record "comments relevant to the individual's drug therapy."[42]

Predictably, some pharmacists opposed this legislation because they felt that any form of mandated counseling infringes upon their professional judgment; others cowered before the specter of increased exposure to legal liability due to what they feel are overly stringent disclosure regulations. In contrast, other pharmacists view the legislation as an affirmation of their professional function, providing an exciting opportunity to exercise their professional judgment, an opportunity for expanded professional service to the American public. Unlike any state or federal legislation that preceded it, Abood and Brushwood declare, OBRA "places public trust in the pharmacist's ability to make decisions that improve the quality of drug therapy and increase the likelihood of good outcomes."[43]

As the legal and ethical standards for patient counseling based upon the pharmacist's professional judgment begin to emerge, the professional disclosure standard for American pharmacists will approach and may even surpass the professional disclosure standard of the prescribing physician. More importantly, as the practice disclosure standard for all health-care professionals in American medical practice moves toward a system of subjective disclosure, practitioners will place greater reliance on patient self-determination, freely providing the information their patients need in making the difficult decisions affecting their health care.

# Ethical Considerations in Pharmacy Communications

As outlined in Chapter 2, the fundamental basis for the pharmacist-patient relationship is trust built upon a solid foundation of shared values. In practice, pharmacists and their patients usually share their values through a delicate web of interpersonal communications. As we have suggested above, however, these communications involve much more than mere "truth-giving." If pharmacists are resolved to strengthen their covenantal relationships with their patients, they will conduct their counseling and all their professional communications in not only a caring manner, but in a manner that respects their patients' claim to autonomy. In so doing, pharmacists can further engage their patients in the process of self-determination, helping them choose their preferred health-care outcomes. The following case studies will provide insight into a number of practice situations, each of which relies not only upon the pharmacist's interpersonal communication skills, but also upon the personal value system of the pharmacist and related ethical principles.

## Considerations when initiating drug therapy

In practice, pharmacists are often confronted by new patients about whom they have little or no information and with whom they have not yet established a relationship of trust. This case explores the obligation of pharmacists to not only fully inform about drug therapy, but also to assure that their patients fully assent to participate in this treatment, thus satisfying both conditions of the so-called "doctrine of informed consent."

### Case 4.1: Assuring Informed Consent

*"Say, what is this drug used for, anyway?"*

Ned Sander is a newly graduated pharmacist who takes pride in his training in clinical pharmacy. The Clinic Pharmacy, an independent professional pharmacy in a physician's clinic building, has an elaborate patient history package in the computer system that he is anxious to use with all his patients. Mrs. Curie, a middle-aged female patient whom Ned has never seen before, approaches the prescription counter. Ned takes her medication history and is struck by the vagueness of her replies. After the interview is completed, Mrs. Curie presents Ned with a new prescription for methotrexate. Ned fills her prescription and provides Mrs. Curie with a rather lengthy list of precautions and possible side effects, making sure she understands how she should take her new medication. Mrs. Curie looks a little dazed after the consultation and suddenly asks Ned, "Say, what is this drug used for, anyway?" Can Ned assume Mrs. Curie did not freely consent to her treatment? Has she been fully informed?

**Commentary:** It is generally agreed among pharmacists that the foundation of the pharmacist-patient relationship is the recognition by society that pharmacy is a profession. This belief, if accepted, leads to a conclusion that pharmacists are thus a "moral community" and that each member of this community understand the duties and obligations placed upon it. Furthermore, members of the community willingly and without prejudice agree to fulfill their professional obligations under all practice conditions. In this case, Ned Sander encounters a basic—perhaps the most basic—moral mandate of professional pharmacy practice: the duty of pharmacists to respect the autonomy of the patient. This particular example may be illustrative of the most frequently encountered ethical dilemma in pharmacy, responding to the seemingly simple question, "What is this drug used for?" It also may be the most difficult to resolve. The right of the patient to make an autonomous choice is the foundation for the concept of informed consent. In the world of law, caregivers who have a duty to inform risk liability by failing to fulfill this duty. In the world of moral philosophy, the duty to inform originates from the principle of respect for autonomy. Unfortunately, both medicine and pharmacy continue to use case law to develop their vision of informing patients, focusing on risk management rather than fulfilling an ethical mandate. Informed consent, which is an integral part of all presurgical procedures, should also be part of the preprescribing procedures of all physicians as well. While many physicians take the time and effort to assure that their patients are informed about their proposed drug therapy, questions such as "What is this drug used for?" may indicate that the patient has not been informed sufficiently or may not have sufficiently understood the information provided by the physician to consent to the use of medications for his or her medical problem.

## Considerations when monitoring drug therapy

Patients occasionally request extra quantities of their prescribed drugs from their pharmacists in anticipation of a vacation or other extended absence. While many maintenance medications pose no legal or ethical problems when dispensed in larger quantities, certain drugs must be monitored carefully by the pharmacist to prevent potential toxicities and other serious side effects, providing a challenge to patient self-determination. The following case presents such a dilemma.

### Case 4.2: Implementing Drug Utilization Review

*"I'll need double the amount this time."*

Mary Jacoby has just completed a drug utilization review on Lethe Rivers, a steady patient and long-time friend of Mary's boss, Al Ebert. Mary became troubled when she saw that Lethe was requesting refills on her prescription for a new benzodiazapene hypnotic with an increasing frequency. Today, as Lethe breezed into the pharmacy for her daily cup of coffee with Mr. Ebert, she stopped by the prescription counter for yet another refill of her hypnotic prescription. "Oh, by the way," Lethe mentioned to Mary, "I'll need double the amount this time." Mary ascertains that Lethe is going on a long cruise and that she has several refills left on her prescription, but is hesitant to provide a large quantity of a drug that she knows can be habit-forming. What is Mary's responsibility to Lethe? Whose values would take precedent in this potential conflict? What part, if any, does Lethe's friendship with Mr. Ebert play in this scenario?

**Commentary:** The role of pharmacists in monitoring drug therapy is widely sanctioned by society. Traditionally, this role has focused on important professional practices such as preventing the dispensing of potentially toxic prescriptions and correcting prescribed physical, chemical, and therapeutic incompatibilities. More recently, pharmacists have begun addressing other drug therapy concerns, some of which may test the boundaries of the pharmacist's duty to be beneficent. The professional practice prerogatives of pharmacists are often enigmatic: they probably exist, and they are probably misunderstood. As pharmacists strive to fully implement the practice of pharmaceutical care, they carve out an increasing number of professional practice prerogatives. Transposing these prerogatives into actions that are founded upon ethical principles remains an engrossing challenge. In this case, Mary Jacoby is considering professional practice prerogatives that center around her evaluation of Lethe's mental stability and her ability to self-determine the proper action. Mary's apparently strong commitment to preventing harm to the patient forces her into an encounter with a number of confounding issues: her relationship to Mr. Ebert, her belief in different value systems, and, most importantly, whether respect for the principle of beneficence has any limits as Mary attempts to fulfill her perceived practice role.

## Considerations involving irrational prescribing

Irrational prescribing by physicians presents one of the most troubling challenges plaguing the profession of pharmacy today. Pharmacists soon learn in practice to not only detect errors, but also to recognize the boundaries of rational, acceptable drug therapy. Pharmacists who detect what in their professional judgment constitutes an unwise or imprudent selection of drugs or dosages face a dilemma: should they quietly fill the prescription as written or intervene with the physician as the tenets of pharmaceutical care require? If they decide to intervene, do they share their concerns with the patient or work out the problem privately with the physician? The following case provides such a dilemma.

### Case 4.3: Establishing Rational Therapy

*"Why do you have to call my doctor?"*

Jack Hancock is an extremely careful, conscientious pharmacist who prides himself in providing a high level of pharmaceutical care to his patients. Today, Jack is troubled. Mrs. Winslow has just presented him with a prescription for a nonnarcotic cough syrup. Jack notes that Dr. John Coxe has written for a subtherapeutic dose, one which could not possibly provide any real therapeutic benefit. After Jack ascertains that the prescription is for Mrs. Winslow, he picks up the phone and dials Dr. Coxe's office and asks to speak to the doctor. Mrs. Winslow overhears Jack's request and breaks in, "Why do you have to call my doctor?" How should Jack respond? Should he share his concerns with Mrs. Winslow or should he attempt to protect Dr. Coxe's reputation? What ethical principles are associated with Jack's decision?

**Commentary:**   Pharmacists have traditionally assumed the mantle of the benevolent servant who protects the patient from the indiscretions of prescribing physicians. Early codes of ethics urged pharmacists to use tact in correcting these indiscretions, shielding the physician from censure and disclosure. The 1994 Code of Ethics for Pharmacists refrains from such specific cautionary declarations, using instead several broad claims for honesty, integrity, and respect. Jack Hancock confronts a situation that has become an integral aspect of professional pharmacy practice over the past three decades: intervening to prevent "irrational prescribing" by physicians. This particular situation is made even more difficult for Jack because the course of medication desired by the prescribing physician would probably not cause any harm; instead, Jack must decide whether Mrs. Winslow would be likely to receive any therapeutic benefit from Dr. Coxe's prescription. Jack now has to decide how to correct this "indiscretion" and to what extent he should share this information with Mrs. Winslow. Jack has already indicated his concern about Mrs. Winslow's prescription and perhaps raised some doubts in her mind. Resolving this dilemma will require Jack to carefully balance his professional practice standards and personal value system with the realities of this practice situation and the needs of both Mrs. Winslow and Dr. Coxe.

## Considerations involving adverse drug reactions

Helping patients avoid adverse drug reactions and monitoring untoward reactions has emerged as one of the most important professional functions pharmacists can perform. Pharmacists are often troubled deciding how much information about side effects and adverse reactions they should share with their patients. Some place a high value upon patient compliance with a prescribed drug regimen and fear too much information will alarm the patient. Others place a high value upon truth-telling and attempt to provide complete disclosure without due regard to compliance. Most pharmacists struggle balancing these two extremes. The following case allows you to engage in this struggle.

## Case 4.4: Monitoring Untoward Reactions

*"This drug makes me feel lousy."*

Reverend Mather, a respected member of the local ministerial association and a renowned marriage counselor, is a long-time patron of Shadyside Pharmacy. His relationships with the professional staff are excellent and in many ways he is a model patient, always cooperating with therapeutic regimens that are suggested for him and seeking additional information about his prescriptions. His personal friendship with pharmacist Lew Diehl is especially strong. A member of his congregation, Lew and his wife have participated in the "marriage encounter" program at the church. As Reverend Mather requests a refill of his prescription for clonidine, Lew asks if he is experiencing any difficulties with the drug. "This drug make me feel lousy!" Reverend Mather exclaims in an uncharacteristic burst of candor. Lew is aware of the strong effect that clonidine can have on the male libido, but feels a little uncomfortable discussing this matter with a man of the cloth. How far should Lew go in eliciting information from Reverend Mather? What roles do personal relationships and personal value systems play in the respect for patient autonomy? Can Lew rely upon a subjective disclosure standard to help him resolve this dilemma?

**Commentary:** Determining the extent to which information about side effects and adverse reactions should be provided to patients is one of the most difficult decisions encountered by practicing pharmacists. It is a practice skill that often seems unattainable to struggling pharmacy students, yet experienced pharmacists somehow get the knack of deciding how much information they need to offer to patients. The Food and Drug Administration (FDA) also recognizes the disparity between what information is known about drugs and what information pharmacists tell patients taking these drugs: the FDA decreed that standardized, written Patient Package Inserts (PPIs) were a possible solution. Proponent and opponents of this governmentally imposed duty to inform continue to debate the merits of PPIs. This case compounds the duty to inform with the additional concerns of human relationships and revealing sensitive, potentially embarrassing medical information: Lew Diehl knows the patient personally; Reverend Mather is his pastor. Now Lew is faced with deciding whether he should proceed with divulging certain information to Reverend Mather about clonidine, its effect on the male libido, the extent to which Reverend Mather's libido is being affected by the clonidine, and exactly how he can collect this information in a dignified and confidential manner. Assuming Lew has cleared this first hurdle, his next ethical choices go beyond the typical clinical benefit-to-risk context. For example, Reverend Mather may ask why Lew did not inform him of the side effects during the initial dispensing of the drug. It would be easy for Lew to slip into a role of "benevolent deception" at this point and become paternalistic. Eventually, Lew will have to address questions of full disclosure and the right of Reverend Mather to determine his own path of action.

## Considerations involving self-medication

The need to self-medicate is deeply ingrained in the American psyche. Indeed, the use of nonprescription drug products is universally recognized by health-care experts as an important characteristic of health behavior. The myriad of nonprescription drug products marketed in the United States provide the consumer with a confusing array of alternatives for self-treatment across a variety of therapeutic categories. Moreover, in recent years, many prescription drugs with demonstrated safety and efficacy have been switched to nonprescription status, increasing further the number of drug products available for autotherapy.

Because pharmacists have the most immediate access to individuals seeking information about drug products and devices used for self-care, they are in a position to influence their patients' decision-making. Indeed, a 1992 California study revealed that 40 per cent of consumers who consulted a pharmacist regarding the use of nonprescription drug products changed their purchasing behavior.[44]

Patients who choose to treat their own complaints often present pharmacists with a bewildering array of queries about over-the-counter products advertised through the media. In counseling these patients, pharmacists must first elicit their real therapeutic needs to determine what—if any—drug product should be recommended. In doing so, they must also sort through the hype and hyperbole of modern marketing while still supporting patients' deeply held, often erroneous, convictions about these products. Unfortunately, some pharmacists practice in settings that do not allow them to weed out suspect or worthless over-the-counter medications and devices from the legitimate products which they could recommend with confidence. The following case presents such a dilemma.

### Case 4.5: Assuring Rational Autotherapy

*"Is this stuff any good for colds?"*

George Markoe is an experienced pharmacist who has recently accepted a position as pharmacist and manager of the flagship outlet of a small midwestern chain operation. George considers his professional practice functions to include maintaining a reasonable selection of over-the-counter drug products that are safe and efficacious for general use. Although part of George's salary is based upon income generated by over-the-counter drugs, George has presented his "drug buyer" with a small list of drug products that do not meet his minimum standards, asking that they be withdrawn and returned for store credit. In today's shipment of store stock he is surprised to find a fairly large floor display of "Relief," a nationally advertised medicated room aerosol intended to relieve the distress caused by head colds. George had already informed his drug buyer that "Relief" was no more than a combination of aromatic chemicals that would have no measurable effect on the symptoms of head colds, especially if diluted by spraying into a large room. As he is studying the attractive display and its engaging advertising slogans, a customer approaches and immediately picks up a can of "Relief." "This is exactly what I am looking for!" exclaims the excited man. "I saw it on television last night. Is this stuff any good for colds?" Should George dissuade this customer from purchasing "Relief" and suggest another product? Should he share his frank opinion of "Relief" with the customer or does the customer have a right to choose his therapy without interference? Should George remove the display of "Relief" and refuse to sell this product?

**Commentary:**  Providing assistance to individuals who attempt to self-medicate to ameliorate personal medical dysfunction is a long-standing and integral part of professional pharmacy practice. The 1981 Code of Ethics of the American Pharmaceutical Association cautioned that pharmacists should not agree to practice under conditions that interfere with their proper exercise of professional judgment. The 1994 Code of Ethics of Pharmacists refrains from such cautions, relying instead on pharmacists' interpretations of fundamental ethical principles of honesty and integrity. In this case, George Markoe is enmeshed in a dilemma that he attempted to avoid. Realizing the consequences of the practical world of medical marketing and advertising, he established a personal standard of practice that includes a carefully drawn evaluation of products that he is willing to make available for self-medication. Unfortunately, his plan is compromised by his institutional venue, resulting in George having to decide whether to shade the truth for the sake of a sale and to mollify his employer or to be honest and continue or even exacerbate the unplanned dilemma.

# Encounters with Other Health Professionals

As established members of the health-care team, pharmacists often find that their professional activities are contingent upon decisions made by physicians, nurses, office secretaries, laboratory technicians, hospital administrators, and other health-care personnel. The need to clarify drug orders, help select the most appropriate drug products, or engage in other activities designed to satisfy patient needs challenges the communication skills of today's pharmacists. The practice philosophy of pharmaceutical care—designing, implementing, and monitoring therapeutic plans that will produce specific therapeutic outcomes in patients—will further challenge pharmacists' interprofessional communication skills.

## Establishing professional communications

Attempting to clarify prescription orders for patients over the telephone poses one of the more trying challenges in professional pharmacy practice. Even the most experienced pharmacy practitioner may be troubled when confronted with the professional and ethical dilemmas that emerge when professional communication is filtered through a third party. The following case presents a typical example of such a dilemma.

### Case 4.6: Clarifying Physician Orders

*"Nurse, may I please speak to the doctor?"*

Louise Baker has established a solid practice of pharmacy over the past five years in Brookline, a suburb of Boston. One of her patients, Stu Craddock, presents Louise with a persistent request to refill his prescription for penicillin. Louise confirms that Stu has been taking his medication as directed and suspects that he may not be benefitting from the prescribed drug therapy. Louise decides to call Dr. Fleming to alert him to the situation. The receptionist who answers explains that Dr. Fleming is very busy and cannot come to the phone. Louise insists that she must speak to the doctor. After a long pause, Dr. Fleming's nurse answers and asks the nature of the call. Louise patiently begins to explain the situation, but is curtly cut off by the nurse. "Oh, you just want a refill. That's all right, go ahead." Louise repeats firmly, "Nurse, may I please speak to the doctor?" How should Louise respond to this situation? Is there a moral mandate for her to assure therapeutic integrity, something beyond her legal need to determine the authenticity of the refill authorization?

**Commentary:** The 1994 Code of Ethics for Pharmacists proclaims that a pharmacist promotes the "good of every patient" in a manner that is caring and compassionate. This extremely broad proclamation of intent, if taken to heart and put into daily practice, often poses some of the more challenging ethical responsibilities in professional practice communications. Attempting to clarify prescription orders for patients over the telephone is a frequent event in pharmacy practice and often one of the most difficult, even for experienced practitioners. Louise Baker is confronted with her perceived professional responsibility to assure that Stu's medical condition requires the refilled medication (thus serving the "good of the patient") and her responsibility to "prevent harm" to Stu (nonmaleficence). Unfortunately, her inquiries are being shunted by the prescribing physician's office staff, preventing her from complying with Stu's request. If the office nurse continues to prevent Louise from speaking to the physician, she will be faced with two choices: refilling the prescription or not refilling it. Complying with Stu's request to refill the prescription may be the most satisfying to all persons involved, except perhaps Louise. Both Stu and the nurse will be relieved since Stu receives the medication he requested and the nurse will be satisfied that her directions were followed. If the prescription is properly annotated with the required refill information, the law will also be satisfied. In the event of any inquiry or clinical complications, Louise could defend her action by saying that the "nurse told me it was okay."

## Validating professional decisions

The American health-care system expects that pharmacists will continue their traditional function as a monitor of therapeutic decision-making, carefully examining prescription orders and validating professional decisions. This function often forces pharmacists to balance the demands of their patients with their real therapeutic needs as well as the therapeutic intention of the physician. The following case illustrates the ethical tension that can arise when these forces are in conflict.

### Case 4.7: Questioning Drug Selection

*"Doc, I really need my pills!"*

Pharmacist Chuck Bullock notes that a local orthopedic surgeon, Dr. Small, routinely prescribes oxycodone for all his patients for relief of pain, in a seemingly casual fashion. While Dr. Small is very conscientious in providing new prescriptions for this powerful drug, Chuck notices that a number of Dr. Small's patients seem to becoming habituated. Some of these patients exhibit signs of the early stages of withdrawal when their prescriptions are not immediately available to be picked up. Today, a highly agitated Tom Quincy, one of Dr. Small's patients, has come into Chuck's pharmacy every two hours asking if his new prescription for his "pain pill" was ready. Chuck replies patiently that Dr. Small has not responded to his repeated telephone calls. Tom explodes, "Doc, I really need my pills!" Chuck feels a moral imperative to confront Dr. Small with his irrational prescribing behavior that is clearly harming his patients. Is Chuck imposing his personal value system on a patient-physician relationship? Should Chuck discuss his concerns with Tom? Should Chuck refuse to fill Tom's prescription and report Dr. Small to the medical board?

**Commentary:** Principles IV and VI of the 1994 Code of Ethics for Pharmacists provide a framework for establishing the relationship between pharmacists and other health providers, using the virtues of honesty, integrity, and respect for values and abilities as the first level for this important foundation. Often, the more immediate relationship between a prescribing physician and dispensing pharmacist becomes strained when a disparity arises concerning the need for a prescribed medication or how that medication is to be used to treat certain conditions. Attempting to honestly respect the values and abilities of the physician may compete with the pharmacist's duty to provide for "the patient's good" as enunciated in Principle II of the 1994 Code. In this case, Chuck Bullock is faced with a practice situation that involves both the patient, Tom, who seeks a "quick fix," and the larger question involving all of Dr. Small's patients who may be subjected to a suspect drug regimen. There is no doubt in Chuck's mind that Tom's pattern of behavior is a manifestation of habituation; Tom's need for his "pain pills" is a matter of grave concern. Unfortunately, the specter of obeying the pharmacy practice act and the easy authorizations of Dr. Small stand in the way of a quick dispensing of the medication, creating an additional moral challenge for Chuck. Does the duty to obey the law override the pharmacist's duty to be caring and compassionate to the patient? As challenging as Tom Quincy's immediate needs are, pharmacist Bullock must still face the troubling and persistent problem of Dr. Small's pattern of drug treatment, especially the use of oxycodone, a highly addictive analgesic. After examining the available options, Chuck realizes the best approach would be to confront Dr. Small and discuss his concerns about his treatment patterns. Although this direct approach may incur unpleasant moments between pharmacist and physician, it is probably the most productive initial avenue.

### Reviewing therapeutic decisions

Pharmacists have dramatically extended the traditional bounds of their professional practice in recent decades, providing important new professional functions that enhance patient care. One of the most challenging of these functions is reviewing the appropriateness of therapeutic decisions of physicians through a formal process of drug utilization review (DUR). The findings from these reviews often require the pharmacist to directly challenge a physician's therapeutic intent when the best interest of the patient demands such intervention. The following case provides practice in dealing with this sensitive issue.

### Case 4.8: Monitoring Drug Utilization

*"Doctor, your patient may be in real danger!"*

Mary Upjohn is a conscientious pharmacist in a small independent pharmacy. Mrs. Lanata, an older lady with cardiac difficulties, presents Mary with a request to refill her prescription order for digoxin. Mary notices that Mrs. Lanata is short of breath and is sweating profusely. Mary asks Mrs. Lanata to sit down and relax and gives her a glass of water. After ascertaining that Mrs. Lanata has been taking her digoxin as prescribed by her physician, she suspects that her prescribed dosage may be incorrect. Mary calls Dr. Withering and explains her concerns. Dr. Withering thanks Mary for her interest, but indicates that he has Mrs. Lanata's congestive heart failure well under control, adding that Mrs. Lanata is "a bit of a hypochondriac" and often calls him about her imaginary complaints. "Just refill her prescription," Dr. Withering says. "I really don't want to see her." "Doctor," Mary blurts out, "your patient may be in real danger!" What is Mary's obligation if she feels Mrs. Lanata is being harmed by Dr. Withering's refusal to see her? Should Mary discuss her concerns with Mrs. Lanata?

**Commentary:**  The medical profession now generally accepts pharmacists' expanded patient care roles, including drug use monitoring and comprehensive patient care management. To meet the challenge of these new roles, pharmacists have had to attain higher levels of clinical practice skills and more assertive communication skills in order to resolve increasingly difficult therapeutic conflicts with physicians. The 1994 Code of Ethics for Pharmacists calls for care, honesty, and the promotion of good for every patient; even without this Code, a pharmacist in professional practice would undoubtedly strive to meet the tenets of a virtuous pharmacist and act decisively to protect the patient. In this case, Mary Upjohn is concerned about the well-being of her patient, Mrs. Lanata, suspecting that a serious problem exists with the dosage of a powerful drug. Rebuffed by Dr. Withering, Mary faces a host of dilemmas, both legal and ethical. The easiest response, simply deferring to Dr. Withering's wishes, may lead to serious, even life-threatening complications for Mrs. Lanata. If Mary decides to discuss her concern with Mrs. Lanata she will certainly be promoting a measure of protection. Mrs. Lanata will be well served, and the principle of nonmaleficence observed, but other problems arise. Does Mary explain to Mrs. Lanata how she came to her decision and how Dr. Withering responded, possibly creating difficult relations between patient and physician? Worse, would such an intervention interfere with or disrupt Mrs. Lanata's drug regimen, causing additional harm?

## Encounters with Other Pharmacists

Pharmacists have enjoyed a long tradition of intraprofessional support for one another in times of stress as well as in times of relative calm. While this tradition has occasionally been marred by the pressures of competition for prescription and other drug-related business, pharmacists have long displayed a strong sense of solidarity, particularly when facing external challenges to their professional prerogatives. The following cases provide practice in dealing with some of these important intraprofessional quandaries.

### Dealing with impaired colleagues

Health professionals who are impaired through substance abuse pose a danger to the patients they serve and a challenge to their interpersonal relationships. These challenges become particularly intense when a pharmacist is attempting to deal with an impaired colleague who is a close personal friend or one's supervisor. The following case presents just such a dilemma.

#### Case 4.9: Assessing Professional Competence

*"Late again? Gus, we have to talk."*

Gus Luhn has been employed as a pharmacist for over thirty years. He has been a dependable member of the professional staff for most of that time. Recently, his attendance has been erratic and the quality of his work has suffered. One of his fellow colleagues, Bill Saunders, has found numerous errors, some of them posing danger to patients. Bill informs the chief pharmacist—and a close friend of Gus's—of his concern, but he refuses to hear any complaints against his old fraternity brother. Yesterday, Bill noticed that Gus was not only unsteady on his feet but took frequent—and long—rest breaks. Bill calls some of Gus's friends and finds that he has a five-year history of abusing alcohol. Today, Gus is supposed to relieve Bill at noon, but shows up two hours late, glassy-eyed and edgy. Bill is understandably concerned, and says, "Late again? Gus, we have to talk." Is there an ethical mandate for Bill to intervene in this situation? Who is affected by Gus's impaired behavior?

**Commentary:** The challenge of monitoring the character and behavior of one's profession is incumbent on all its members, from novice students to experienced practitioners. Often, the misbehavior or unworthy attitude of a colleague is a matter of degree rather than substance; nevertheless, the need to meet professional pharmacy practice standards, especially regarding professional competence, is a paramount obligation for every member of the pharmacy profession. Professional and personal behavior attitudes ingrained during the earliest periods of professional development are critical to lifelong practice patterns and generally establish the foundation for all professional relationships, including intraprofessional relationships. In this case, Bill Saunders is concerned with the behavior of his colleague, Gus, but meets resistance as he attempts to question—and perhaps correct—the troubling situation. There is no question that pharmacists have a moral obligation to promote the good of every patient. In discharging this duty, they should, at a minimum, at least prevent any harm. Ordinarily, pharmacists feel they meet this obligation by screening prescribed medications for problems or providing expert information to help their patients make optimal use of medicines for autotherapy. Judging the worthiness of actions of pharmacist colleagues is not a common occurrence, yet as this case demonstrates, denying this challenge may be disastrous for the patient. Complicating this case is the long-standing fraternal relationship between the chief pharmacist and Gus. Bill wonders if the blind devotion exhibited by the chief pharmacist is not a carryover attitude ingrained during his college years, one that never progressed beyond the initial level of personal commitment. If Bill persists, he may not only injure his relationship with Gus, but his relationships among other colleagues at his practice site. Ultimately, Bill will have to decide whether his duty to protect patients is greater than his call to respect the ability and judgment of the chief pharmacist.

## Maintaining continuity of patient care

Patients have a right to the same high level of professional care each time they receive pharmaceutical services. Whether patients choose to be served by two pharmacists operating an independent office practice or by a dozen or more pharmacists practicing in a hospital or a large chain setting, they should expect continuity in both the nature and the extent of professional services they receive. The following case illustrates what can happen when that continuity is breached.

## Case 4.10: Preserving Patient Confidence

*"The other pharmacist never told me that!"*

Jim Shinn, a recent graduate of a prestigious college of pharmacy in the east, has just accepted a position at Sloan's Pharmacy in Indianapolis. Jim is eager to share his knowledge of drugs with his patients, and is careful to provide them with detailed counseling. Mrs. Nation presents Jim with a request to refill her prescription for diazepam. Jim refills the prescription and begins to counsel Mrs. Nation about the adverse effects she might experience while taking this drug. He concludes his remarks by cautioning Mrs. Nation to avoid drinking alcoholic beverages one hour before or after her dose of diazepam. "Why, what could happen?" Mrs. Nation asks, visibly shaken. Jim explains that Mrs. Nation could become seriously ill. "The other pharmacist never told me that!" Should Jim cover for Mr. Sloan, preserving Mrs. Nation's confidence in him? Should Jim soften his warning or reaffirm it? What is Jim's obligation to Mr. Sloan in this situation?

**Commentary:** While the 1994 Code of Ethics for Pharmacists makes only an oblique reference about behavioral relationships among pharmacists, earlier codes included direct, specific ethical guidelines regulating such behavior. The 1952 APhA Code of Ethics encouraged pharmacists to adopt many behaviors: they were enjoined to perfect and enlarge their professional knowledge, attract youth of good character into the profession, keep their reputation in the public esteem, avoid activities that bring discredit to the profession, expose corrupt or dishonest members of the profession, aid any fellow pharmacist that seeks help, meet obligations promptly, and be proud to display their name in their place of practice. Principle VI of the 1994 Code of Ethics for Pharmacists simply declares that a pharmacist "respects the values and abilities of colleagues and other health professionals." This redefinition and refocus of intraprofessional ethical behavior clearly emphasizes the foundation of pharmaceutical care, the total commitment of pharmacists to patient care. Interpreting and implementing Principle VI of the 1994 Code remains a formidable challenge for practicing pharmacists, especially as they place the respect for the values and abilities of colleagues in the context of honesty, integrity, and covenantal relationships with patients. In this case, Jim Shinn is being prompted to reveal information about his colleague, Mr. Sloan, that might impugn his professional reputation or cast discredit upon him. Mrs. Nation understands that something is amiss and seeks comfort. Unfortunately for Jim, two separate duties are starting to converge: loyalty and respect toward a colleague and veracity in providing professional services. Jim must sort out the facts, arrange them in concert with his personal value system, and select a course of action. To waffle and provide a softened "nonanswer" to Mrs. Nation may avoid embarrassment to the pharmacy staff, but this strategy would also provide less than an honest reply. Yet, since Mrs. Nation has not suffered any physical harm up to this point, is complete honesty the overriding moral principle?

## Reconciling perceived discrepancies

Because patients depend upon their prescription drugs to maintain their health or cure their diseases, they often develop a deep interest in the continuity of their drug therapy. Any slight departure from the expected shape, color, or size of their prescription drug products can not only create anxiety in the mind of these patients, but can undermine the relationship of trust between patient and pharmacist. The following case illustrates how a seemingly minor modification in a patient's drug therapy can affect this trust.

### Case 4.11: Defending Drug Product Selection

*"My refill looks different. Do I have the right drug?"*

Pharmacist Chuck Heinitsh works in a high-volume chain pharmacy in a large eastern city. His manager, Mr. Bedford, has just received a communication from the corporate office informing him that from now on the chain will be purchasing its generic drug line from a different manufacturer. Both Chuck and Mr. Bedford have confidence in the new manufacturer, but notice that many of the solid dosage forms differ in size, shape, or color from the generic drug line they had been dispensing. Today, Chuck receives a telephone call from Ted Janeway asking him to refill his generic prescription for hydrochlorothiazide and have it delivered. Later that afternoon, Mr. Janeway calls the pharmacy and asks to speak to "that pharmacist who was working this morning." Chuck is a little wary as he picks up the telephone, but says brightly, "This is the pharmacist. May I help you?" "This is Mr. Janeway" an agitated voice replies. "My refill looks different. Do I have the right drug?" What is the ethical dilemma in this case? How can Chuck regain Mr. Janeway's confidence?

Commentary: As recent Gallup Polls have affirmed, pharmacists have long enjoyed an enviable reputation throughout all strata of American society for their honesty and trustworthiness. Maintaining this level of trust depends on the integrity of relationships developed during all aspects of professional pharmacy practice, none of which are more important than individual patient counseling. Principle I of the 1994 Code of Ethics for Pharmacists establishes the foundation of the pharmacist-patient relationship as covenantal, and warns of the necessity of maintaining trust in this relationship. With the current profusion of multisource drug products, this case demonstrates not only the need to assure sufficient communication between the pharmacist and the patient at all times, but also the need for this communication to take place at the right time, in this case, before the dispensing of the prescribed medication. The color, shape, and manufacturer of dosage forms may appear trivial to the pharmacist at times, but may be crucial in maintaining patient confidence. Chuck Heinitsh is now probably wishing he had taken the time earlier to be more complete in his counseling of Mr. Janeway. Nevertheless, Chuck now has to balance two sets of needs: those of Mr. Janeway and those needed to restore a confident pharmacist-patient relationship.

## Encounters with the General Public

The community pharmacist enjoys a long tradition of service to the public. No other health-care practitioner is so readily accessible to the public for advice and counseling on drug-related issues, simple first-aid procedures, and other issues related to individual and public health. During a typical day, a community pharmacist might provide advice on a wide variety of over-the-counter drugs and personal care items, urge a workman with a deep puncture wound to seek immediate medical attention rather than self-medicate, consult with the local board of health about a new immunization program, speak to a group of school children on drug abuse, or appear on a local radio talk-show with a physician to discuss possible treatments for an outbreak of flu. This willingness to provide compassionate, reliable advice is reflected by recent public opinion polls that attest to the trust and confidence the public places in their pharmacists. The following cases discuss the sort of dilemmas that arise when this public image of trust is compromised.

## Establishing a professional image

Like other health professionals, pharmacists cherish the high professional status that is conferred upon them by the public. Unfortunately, competitive pressures and other internal and external forces may tempt some pharmacists to seek an unfair advantage over their colleagues through the use of deceptive advertising. By implying that other pharmacists are financially exploiting their patients through high prescription prices or making claims of professional superiority that cannot be verified, these pharmacists risk undermining their professional image by engaging in this type of deception. The following case provides an illustration of this professional issue.

### Case 4.12: Advertising Professional Services

#### *"PRESCRIPTIONS ACCURATELY COMPOUNDED!"*

Bill Thompson is the proud new owner of a professional pharmacy specializing in compounding prescriptions. He is eager to establish a loyal clientele who would benefit from his special professional service. Bill decides to engage a local advertising agency to develop a campaign to alert both physicians and the public. A few weeks later, the head of Hopkins Advertising arrives with a portfolio of advertising layouts he hopes Bill will adopt. "PRESCRIPTIONS ACCURATELY COMPOUND-ED!" the headline of one ad proclaims boldly. "We use only the freshest ingredients in our prescriptions, which we fill exactly to your doctor's specifications." "Well, what do you think?" Mr. Hopkins asks proudly. Bill sees no factual error in the copy, but somehow feels it is not really "professional." What might be causing Bill's uneasiness? To what extent is advertising professional services affected by ethical principles?

**Commentary:** Earlier codes of ethics in American pharmacy alerted pharmacists to potential difficulties caused by certain types of public proclamations or solicitations. The 1952 APhA Code of Ethics proclaimed that the ethical pharmacist "does not imitate labels" of his competitors or take "unfair advantage" of their commercial success. The 1969 Code stated a pharmacist "should not solicit professional practice by means of advertising." More recently, the Federal Trade Commission (FTC) has ruled such bans on advertising to be in conflict with the public's right to have this kind of information. As a result, pharmacy and other professions have deleted such prohibitions from their codes of ethics. Nevertheless, some types of advertising may not be consistent with reasonable ethical standards, and Bill Thompson is disturbed by Mr. Hopkin's proposed advertising campaign. Realizing that the proffered advertising copy has no factual error, seems direct to the point, and is, in fact, the kind of information the FTC believes the public has the right to access, Bill could rationalize the appropriateness of the copy upon his correlative duty to provide such access. After all, the statement is true: Bill prides himself on accuracy and fastidiously controls compounding stock to ensure freshness. Bill may be overlooking some consequences that could result from faulty or imperfect public interpretation of the advertisement. For example, some of the public may believe there are pharmacists who compound prescriptions inaccurately or use stale or outdated ingredients. Bill certainly did not intend to send this message in his advertising; nevertheless, this sort of advertising certainly does not show "respect for the values and abilities of colleagues."

## Championing the cause of public health

One often overlooked aspect of pharmacists' professional function is their advocacy of public health concerns. Over the years, pharmacists have demonstrated their concern for important public health issues in a variety of ways from volunteering in a mass community immunization program to screening people for diabetes or high blood pressure. Pharmacists also encounter many situations where their specialized knowledge of drug products can safeguard the unwary public from the dangers of unreliable or untested therapies, as the following case illustrates.

### Case 4.13: Monitoring Questionable Products

*"Do you carry DMSO?"*

Ed Kendall, an elderly man with advanced arthritis, enters the Ingalls Pharmacy slowly. He is obviously experiencing great pain as he scans the shelves in the analgesic section.

Pharmacist Jack Ingalls approaches Mr. Kendall and asks
how he can help him. "I've tried everything for this arthritis
of mine," Mr. Kendall explains wearily. "The drugs my doctor
have prescribed for me no longer control my pain, and I don't
want to take higher doses or any narcotics." Jack reviews Mr.
Kendall's drug therapy, but sees no immediate alternative. He
offers to call Mr. Kendall's physician to discuss his problem,
but Mr. Kendall shakes his head. "My doctor has done everything he could do," he replies. "Do you carry DMSO?" Jack
realizes that he has a small container of dimethyl sulfoxide in
stock as part of the solvents carried in the pharmacy and also
understands the off-label use for arthritic pain that has developed over the last several years. However, he believes such use
of DMSO is dangerous and not likely to provide long-term
benefits to the patient. What is Jack's responsibility to Mr.
Kendall? When does patient benefit surpass potential risk?

**Commentary:** The 1994 Code of Ethics for Pharmacists states
that pharmacists "assist individuals in making the best use of their
medications," an apparently unbounded promise to assist patients
in the use of all their medications, regardless of source, whether
prescribed or not. Conventional medical practices are ordinarily
considered those which have been tried, tested, and ultimately approved by recognized medical and legal authorities. From the
patient's viewpoint, however, medications may include a wide variety of substances, such as folk remedies, naturally occurring products, or complex mixtures of inorganic or organic chemicals, some
of which are often labeled as untested for safety or considered unreliable in their therapeutic action. Pharmacists who accept the duty
to assist patients with all their medications will invariably encounter situations that will pit these conflicting viewpoints, prompting
difficult decisions that are usually centered on balancing a potential risk to the patient with a perceived possible benefit. In this
case, Mr. Kendall, exasperated by his traditional arthritic therapy,
inquires about the use of a medication that has not been approved
for human use. Jack Ingalls, while sympathetic to Mr. Kendall, has
doubt about the efficacy of DMSO in treating arthritis as well as
the potential toxicity of its use. Furthermore, he notices that although DMSO is not a legend drug, the bottle is clearly labeled (in
red) "to be used or sold for manufacturing or veterinary purposes
only." Jim could decide that ultimately the decision to use this
drug lies with the patient, and through a well-conceived disclosure
of all pertinent information, allow Mr. Kendall to make his own de-

cision about its use. Such an approach would not obviate Jim's feelings of concern about the benefits of extended use of DMSO or its possible untoward side effects, but it does provide respect for the patient's right of self-determination, one of the basic moral principles of professional pharmacy practice.

## Extending professional services to the public

Finally, pharmacists have traditionally displayed a strong sense of altruism in their dealings with the public. This is reflected in a long-standing, common commitment among pharmacists to provide professional services to their patients. Examples of this behavior range from extending credit to patients requiring immediate drug therapy to providing small quantities of medicine from an expired prescription when the physician cannot be reached in order to maintain needed drug therapy. While performing compassionate acts in the practice of pharmacy is laudable, they should be accomplished within a defensible framework of personal values. The following case provides an opportunity to challenge your personal value framework.

### Case 4.14: Performing Compassionate Acts

*"You need a prescription for this, but . . ."*

Joe Roberts prides himself on providing a caring response to the needs of his patients. Late one evening, just before closing, Paul Link enters Joe's pharmacy with a concerned expression on his face. "My wife and I are out of town on vacation and I've forgotten my blood-thinner pills," Paul explains. Joe ascertains that Paul has been taking his dicumarol properly for the past fourteen months and has just received a new prescription for the drug from his physician following a routine checkup. Joe attempts to contact both his pharmacist and his physician back home without success. Joe realizes that Paul is in no immediate medical danger, but understands that interruption of the dicumarol therapy may alter his prothrombin time, necessitating a long and rather costly titration procedure. Joe also realizes that if Paul does not continue his dicumarol therapy he may develop potentially dangerous clotting episodes. Joe hesitates briefly and then says, "You need a prescription for this, but . . ." His voice trails off as he considers his quandary. What should Joe do in this case? Do Paul's medical needs supersede Joe's legal obligation? Does Joe have a professional obligation to come to Paul's assistance? Does Joe possess the clinical expertise to come to Paul's assistance?

**Commentary:** The pharmacist-patient relationship, like all relationships between health-care professionals and their patients, is the ultimate foundation for developing professional practice behavior, especially in response to patient requests. Pharmacists and their patients establish these relationships during the usual and ordinary course of providing and receiving pharmacy services. There are times, however, when the existence of a pharmacist-patient relationship may not be apparent to either person, or is assumed to exist by one party but not the other. Whether the relationship is covenantal, as proposed by the 1994 Code of Ethics for Pharmacists, or more narrowly viewed as a social contract, there needs to be sufficient awareness by both patient and pharmacist about the viability of the foundation of their relationship. This case seems simple, yet can become complex if the pharmacist guides his action based upon the tenets of a true, traditional pharmacist-patient relationship rather than an unique request for assistance from a stranger. When does the pharmacist-patient relationship begin and under what conditions? If Joe Roberts has a complete commitment to his patients, he should provide professional services following the full range of ethical values. Most pharmacists would believe that Joe should provide a limited quantity of the needed medication to Paul, relying upon a professional prerogative that supersedes all legal restraints. Joe could defend this action to himself, his peers, and perhaps the law, on the grounds of providing good for the patient. In this instance, good for the patient refers to the means to sustain a complex, vital medical regimen of therapy.

## Concluding Remarks

In this chapter we have seen that pharmacists can encounter a wide array of ethical dilemmas in their communications with their patients, with other health-care providers, and with other pharmacists. Pharmacists often must decide whether they should filter, enhance, or otherwise modify these communications in order to improve patient care. More importantly, as a moral disclosure standard becomes an accepted tenet of professional pharmacy practice, pharmacists will need to carefully examine their personal value systems to ensure that their professional communications meet the independent informational needs of their patients.

## Study Questions

4.1 Make a list of values that are important to you in professional practice communications. Are these learned values?

4.2 How do pharmacists determine the informational needs of patients? Describe the process.

4.3 Upon what authority does the moral disclosure standard depend?

## Situations for Analysis

4.1 An oncology surgeon with a national reputation practices at a large university hospital. He persists in treating his patients with large doses of a highly specialized blood fraction that he feels speeds healing time although clinical studies do not support this claim. This year, the use of this drug product by this single physician will add nearly $500,000 to the pharmacy department's budget. As the pharmacy representative to the hospital's pharmacy and therapeutics committee, you are asked by the director of pharmacy to remove this product from the hospital formulary.

4.2 A patient presents you with a prescription container from a rival pharmacy and asks you to refill it. You dial the number of the other pharmacy and ask to speak with the pharmacist. After identifying yourself you ask for the prescription information and are told curtly, "We don't give out copies!"

4.3 A doctor telephones a prescription for a powerful tranquilizer, but directs you to label the prescription with the name of a mild sedative because the patient is "frightened by the idea of taking tranquilizers." The drug prescribed is the only effective therapy for this condition. Your state pharmacy practice act includes a strong prohibition against mislabeling.

4.4 A patient with a history of anxiety reactions and hypochondriacal complaints presents the pharmacist with a prescription for

40 5-mg tablets of diazepam. The pharmacist believes that taking anxiolytics is a sign of personal weakness and that those who suffer from anxiety should "snap out of it." To dissuade people from taking tranquilizers, the pharmacist routinely tells such patients alarming stories of dependence, and does with this patient, who leaves the pharmacy in a clearly agitated state.

# References

1. Joseph W. England, ed., *The First Century of the Philadelphia College of Pharmacy, 1821-1921* (Philadelphia: By the College, 1922), p. 72. Also see *Formulae for the Preparation of Eight Patent Medicines, Adopted by the Philadelphia College of Pharmacy, May 4th, 1824* (Philadelphia: Solomon W. Conrad, 1824).

2. Edward Parrish, "Ethical Analysis," *Proceedings of the American Pharmaceutical Association 6* (1857), p. 149.

3. Edward Parrish, *A Treatise on Pharmacy*, 4th ed., edited by Thomas S. Wiegand (Philadelphia: Henry C. Lea, 1874), p. 902. "Even in conversation with the least intelligent," Parrish suggested, the pharmacist should "remove the rough edges of their ignorance, by well-directed remarks and explanations." *Ibid.*

4. "The nineteenth century ended with the two professions having found a *modus vivendi* whose details had to be repeatedly spelled out," pharmacy historian David L. Cowen has concluded. "Each was aware of its own prerogatives, and each was determined to protect its own turf." See David L. Cowen, "Changing Relationships Between Pharmacists and Physicians," *American Journal of Hospital Pharmacy 49*:11 (November, 1992), p. 2717.

5. See Charles H. LaWall, "Pharmaceutical Ethics: A Historical Review of the Subject with Examples of Codes Adopted or Suggested at Different Periods, Together with a Suggested Code for Adoption by Present-Day Associations," *Journal of the American Pharmaceutical Association 10*:11 (November, 1921), pp. 898 and 901. The Philadelphia code characterized pharmacists' errors as arising from one of four sources: from the "imperfect handwriting" of physicians, from "imperfect abbreviations" for various synonyms of drugs in use, from "the confusion which even in the best regulated establishments may sometimes occur, arising from press of business," and from "deficient knowledge and ability" of either pharmacists or their assistants. Interestingly, physicians were asked to make a "distinction between an error made by a younger assistant accidentally engaged, and a case of culpable ignorance or carelessness in the superior."

6. Wilbur L. Scoville, *The Art of Compounding*, 4th ed. (Philadelphia: P. Blakiston's Son & Co., 1914), p. 5. This wording persisted until the eighth edition in 1951, tempered only by time and progress. "Much of the need for secrecy that surrounded the nature and properties of medicines in former times has disappeared with the advent of new highly efficient

drugs and a general rise in the intelligence of the laity." See Glenn L. Jenkins, Don E. Francke, Edward A. Brecht, and Glen J. Sperandio, *Scoville's The Art of Compounding*, 8th ed. (Philadelphia: The Blakiston Company, 1951), pp. 1-2.

7. "Code of Ethics of the American Pharmaceutical Association (Adopted August 17, 1922)," *Journal of the American Pharmaceutical Association* *11*:9 (September, 1922), p. 729; and "Code of Ethics of the American Pharmaceutical Association," *Journal of the American Pharmaceutical Association* (Practical Pharmacy Edition) *13*:10 (October, 1952), p. 722.

8. Henry V. Arny and Robert P. Fischelis, *Principles of Pharmacy*, 4th ed. (Philadelphia: W. B. Saunders Company, 1937), p. 1055. Reflecting the standards of the 1922 APhA Code, Arny and Fischelis offered an additional "case study" to their students: "A nervous woman wants to know what a certain prescription she holds in her hand is good for and what are its constituents. The tactful pharmacist responds that these are questions which the physician who wrote the prescription is alone permitted to answer, and expresses his willingness to place the lady in telephonic connection with the doctor. His kindly offer is declined." *Ibid.*

9. William J. Husa, *Pharmaceutical Dispensing*, 4th ed. [Easton, Pennsylvania: Mack Printing Co.], 1951, p. 698.

10. "If a customer asks what disease a prescription is for, the pharmacist can compliment him on the interest he takes in his health," Husa recommended in 1947. "Then he can add, 'Your physician gave it to you for your relief and benefit; you must place yourself in his care.'" See William J. Husa, *Pharmaceutical Dispensing*, 3rd ed. (Easton, Pennsylvania: Mack Printing Company, 1947), p. 679.

11. Glenn L. Jenkins, Glen J. Sperandio, and Clifton J. Latiolais, *Clinical Pharmacy: A Text for Dispensing* (New York: McGraw-Hill Book Company, 1966), p. 39. The term "clinical pharmacy" was described as "the most appropriate designation for the professional applications of the pharmacist in his dealings with the public," *Ibid.*, p. v.

12. *Ibid.*, p. 37.

13. Eric W. Martin, ed. *Dispensing of Medication*, 7th ed. (Easton, Pennsylvania: Mack Publishing Company, 1971), p. 29. The essentially mercantile attitude clouding early clinical pharmacy practice is reflected in the next paragraph: "While delivering the prescription, the pharmacist may also suggest related health needs and accessories which the patient will need. . . . Such suggestions may save the patient a return trip and, at the same time, increase pharmacy sales." *Ibid.*, pp. 29 and 31.

14. [Forrest T. Patterson,] "In Summary . . . Workshop Discussions," *Journal of the American Pharmaceutical Association* NS8:3 (March, 1968), pp. 143-44. Participants hedged upon full disclosure, however, noting that "it would not be necessary to make the patient aware of the therapeutic effect of a prescribed drug." *Ibid.*, p. 143.

15. Kenneth S. Griswold, "Report of the Judicial Board," *Journal of the American Pharmaceutical Association* NS8:7 (July, 1968), pp. 355-56. Members of the Judicial Board volunteered to attend state and local association meetings to discuss the proposed Code. Griswold also submitted the proposed Code to a special meeting of the APhA House of Delegates in Chicago, November 24-25, 1968. See "Members Comments Sought on Proposed Code," *APhA Newsletter 7*:13 (July 13, 1968), p. 1; and Kenneth S. Griswold, "Report of the Judicial Board," *Journal of*

*the American Pharmaceutical Association NS9*:7 (July, 1969), p. 329.

16. The proposed Code was modified to broaden the scope of Section 5 and make clear that "transactions which may result in financial or other exploitation of the patient . . . are deemed unethical." By September, 1969, the new Code had been approved by the membership. See "Proposed APhA Code of Ethics," *APhA Election Bulletin*, July 21, 1969, p. [6]; and "Whitten Elected APhA President, Parks Chosen As Vice President," *APhA Newsletter 8*:18 (September, 1969), p. 1.

17. "Legal Considerations in Adopting and Enforcing a Profession-Wide Code of Ethics," memorandum from Ms. Patricia Schultheiss to Dr. John A. Gans, American Pharmaceutical Association, November 15, 1989.

18. "Code of Ethics for Pharmacists," approved by the Board of Trustees of the American Pharmaceutical Association, September, 1993. The new Code was approved by the membership of the Association on October 27, 1994.

19. *Ibid.*, Section III.

20. "Statement on a Patient's Bill of Rights," in André L. Lee and Godfrey Jacobs, "Workshop Airs Patients' Rights," *Hospitals 47*:4 (February 16, 1973), p. 41. The Bill of Rights included the right to information about treatment and prognosis, the right to refuse treatment, the right to privacy, the right to knowledge about human experimentation, and the right to considerate and respectful care. A revision of the Bill of Rights was approved by the American Hospital Association's Board of Trustees on October 21, 1992 (see Appendix B).

21. Robert M. Veatch, "The Pharmacist and the Patients' Rights Movement," *U.S. Pharmacist 4*:1 (January, 1979), p. 94.

22. "Minimum Standard for Pharmacies in Institutions," *American Journal of Hospital Pharmacy 34*:12 (December, 1977), p. 1357. "This is particularly important for ambulant and discharge patients," the Standard continued. "These patient education activities shall be coordinated with the nursing and medical staffs and patient education department (if any.)"

23. Samuel H. Kalman and John F. Schlegel, "Standards of Practice for the Profession of Pharmacy," *American Pharmacy NS19*:3 (March, 1979), pp. 134, 142-44. To meet these standards of practice, the pharmacist "clarifies patient's understanding of dosage; integrates drug-related with patient-related information; advises patient of potential drug-related conditions; refers patient to other health care resources; monitors and evaluates therapeutic response of patient; reviews and/or seeks additional drug-related information." *Ibid.*, p. 142.

24. Thomas F. McMahon, "The Professional's Responsibility," *Journal of the American Pharmaceutical Association NS12*:7 (July, 1972), pp. 358, 359.

25. Study Commission on Pharmacy, *Pharmacists for the Future: The Report of the Study Commission on Pharmacy* (Bethesda, Maryland: Health Administration Press, 1975), pp. 139-40 and 99-100. "Pharmacy knowledge is disseminated to physicians, pharmacists, and other health professionals and to the general public to the end that drug knowledge and products may contribute to the health of individuals and the welfare of society," the Commission concluded. *Ibid.*, p. 140.

26. "Statement on Pharmacist-Conducted Patient Counseling," *American Journal of Hospital Pharmacy 33*:1 (July, 1976), pp. 644-45. "It is well-

documented that safe and effective drug therapy most frequently oc-
curs when patients are well-informed about medications and their use,"
the Statement concluded. "Knowledgeable patients exhibit increased
compliance with drug regimens, resulting in improved therapeutic outcomes."

27. Dorothy L. Smith, "Patient Compliance with Medication Regimens,"
    *Drug Intelligence and Clinical Pharmacy 10*:7 (July, 1976), p. 386. Re-
    ports of drug misuse have appeared in the medical literature since 1946.
    See Darrell R. Newcomer and Roger W. Anderson, "Effectiveness of a
    Combined Drug Self-Administration and Patient Teaching Program,"
    *ibid. 8*:6 (June, 1974), p. 374.
28. See, for example, Marshall H. Becker and Lois A. Maiman,
    "Sociobehavioral Determinants of Compliance with Health and Medi-
    cal Care Recommendations," *Medical Care 13*:1 (January, 1975), pp. 10-
    24.
29. John P. Kirscht and Irwin M. Rosenstock, "Patients' Problems in Fol-
    lowing Recommendations of Health Experts," in George C. Stone,
    Frances Cohen, and Nancy E. Adler, eds., *Health Psychology—A Hand-
    book* (San Francisco: Jossey-Bass, 1979), p. 199.
30. See, for example, Amy K. Lezberg and David A. Fedo, "Communica-
    tion Skills and Pharmacy Education: A Case Study," *American Journal
    of Pharmaceutical Education 44*:3 (August, 1980), p. 257. "There is
    scarcely a pharmacy institution in the United States that has not added,
    or is not in the process of adding, a communications component to its
    undergraduate curriculum," Lezberg and Fedo asserted.
31. Paul J. Matte, Jr., "The Community Pharmacist—Prescriptions, Pro-
    prietaries and Legal Problems," *Journal of the American Pharmaceutical
    Association NS10*:8 (August, 1970), p. 450.
32. David A. Kessler, "Communicating With Patients About Their Medi-
    cations," *The New England Journal of Medicine 325*:23 (December 5,
    1991), pp. 1650-52.
33. Brenda Raffath, "Does the Pharmacist Have a Duty to Warn Patients
    of a Prescription Medication's Potential Risks or Danger," *The Journal
    of Pharmacy & Law 1*:1 (1992), p. 73.
34. In their discussion of pharmacists' legal liability for failure to perform
    expanded responsibilities associated with delivering pharmaceutical care,
    Abood and Brushwood note that the pharmacist has a *legal* duty to
    monitor and intervene only if 1) the pharmacist-patient relationship
    gives rise to an expanded duty, 2) if harm to the patient is "reasonably
    foreseeable" to the pharmacist, and 3) if "public health concerns" (such
    as increasing health care costs and diminished public confidence in phy-
    sicians) favor recognizing such an expanded duty. See Richard R. Abood
    and David B. Brushwood, *Pharmacy Practice and the Law*, 3rd ed.
    (Gaithersburg, Maryland: Aspen Publishers, Inc., 2001), pp. 330-33.
35. Tom L. Beauchamp and James F. Childress, *Principles of Biomedical
    Ethics*, 5th ed. (New York and Oxford: Oxford University Press, 2001),
    pp. 81-82. Beauchamp and Childress discuss the standards of disclosure
    within the context of the principle of respect for autonomy.
36. *Ibid.*
37. The patient should be provided with information that a reasonable per-
    son in the patient's circumstances "would find relevant and could rea-
    sonably be expected to assimilate," Beauchamp and Childress argue.

"In this way the moral requirement to respect autonomy is translated into a reasonable person standards of disclosure." *Ibid.*, p. 89.

38. Ruth R. Fadden and Tom L. Beauchamp, *A History and Theory of Informed Consent* (New York and Oxford: Oxford University Press, 1986), p. 32.

39. *Ibid.*, pp. 35-36. The authors state that "physicians would not be expected under the standard to do more than make a reasonable effort to determine their patients' desires," yet note that "it cannot be made precise how much effort would be deemed 'reasonable' under any given circumstance."

40. Tom L. Beauchamp and James F. Childress, *Principles of Biomedical Ethics*, 5th ed. (New York and Oxford: Oxford University Press, 2001), pp. 81-82. Beauchamp and Childress discuss the standards of disclosure for physicians within the context of the principle of respect for autonomy.

41. Public Law No. 101-508, §4206, "Medicare Provider Agreements Assuring the Implementation of a Patient's Right to Participate in and Direct Health Care Decisions Affecting the Patient," *United States Code Congressional and Administrative News, 101st Congress, Second Session, 1990* (St. Paul, Minnesota: West Publishing Company, 1991), Vol. 2, 104 Stat. 1388, 115-16 (1990). This section, popularly referred to as the "Patient Self-Determination Act of 1990," amends provisions of the Social Security Act regarding Medicare and Medicaid.

42. Public Law No. 101-508, §4401, "Reimbursement for Prescribed Drugs," *United States Code Congressional and Administrative News, 101st Congress, Second Session, 1990* (St. Paul, Minnesota: West Publishing Company, 1991), Vol. 2, 104 Stat. 1388, 152-53 (1990).

43. See, for example, Dianne M. Tharp, "Ostriches Beware: The New Standard of Practice," *Drug Store News for the Pharmacist 2*:6 (June 22, 1992), p. 4; David Brushwood, "No Liability Despite State Board Counseling Mandate," *NABP Newsletter 20*:10 (November-December, 1991), p. 108; and Abood and Brushwood, *Pharmacy Practice and the Law* (n. 34), p. 239. Although patients can waive the right to be counseled about their drug therapy, OBRA contemplates an "informed right" to counseling, Abood and Brushwood note. Clerks who ask "You don't want to talk to the pharmacist, do you?" do not provide patients with the type of informed choice that Congress anticipated. *Ibid.*, p. 244.

44. Michael B. Nichol, Jeffrey S. McCombs, Kathleen A. Johnson, Shirlynn Spacapan, and David A. Sclar, "The Effects of Consultation on Over-the-Counter Medication Purchasing Decisions," *Medical Care 30*:11 (November, 1992), p. 1001. The authors note that approximately 15 per cent of the patients in their study purchased no over-the-counter product after receiving a pharmacist's consultation.

## Suggested Readings

Brushwood, David B. "Legal Expectations of Expanded Pharmacy Practice." *Wisconsin Pharmacist* [*60*:6] (October, 1991), pp. 5-7.

Kilwein, J[ohn] H. "Commentary: Disguising Morals as Medicine." *Journal of Clinical Pharmacy and Therapeutics 13* (1988), pp. 179-81.

Young, James Harvey. *American Self-Dosage Medicines: An Historical Perspective*. Lawrence, Kansas: Coronado Press, 1974.

# CHAPTER 5

# ETHICAL CONSIDERATIONS IN DRUG DISTRIBUTION

Up to this point, we have been focusing upon pharmacists' responses to ethical challenges to their professional practice. We have also traced the rise of the consumerism movement, which set the stage for countless (and often heated) dialogues over the prescription counter about the price and quality of drug products. In recent years, these dialogues have taken on a broader, even national character.

In April 1993, for example, the National People's Action, a Chicago-based consumer group representing over 300 local consumer organizations, attempted to take over the Washington offices of the Pharmaceutical Manufacturers Association to protest the soaring costs of prescription drugs.[1] In September, the Board of Trustees of the American Pharmaceutical Association (APhA) endorsed the Coordinated Care Network of PAID Prescriptions, Inc., a managed care plan to compensate pharmacists for their cognitive professional services, generating a firestorm of protest across the pharmaceutical community.[2] In October, in an unusual display of solidarity, a group of drugstore chains and independent pharmacies filed suit in federal court charging seven of the largest drug manufacturers with a wide range of violations of federal antitrust laws, including price discrimination and price-fixing.[3] In September 1999, the Federal Trade Commission began investigating "sweetheart deals" between brand-name pharmaceutical manufacturers and manufacturers of their generic counterparts, reducing the promise of more widely available generic drugs.[4] These examples underscore the tortuous changes affecting the American drug distribution system, many of which have profound ethical implications. Are these changes an isolated phenomenon or do they reflect the expansion of the American drug distribution system?

## Expansion of the drug distribution system

At the turn of the century, most urban Americans obtained their drugs and health-care needs from the corner drugstore; their rural neighbors purchased their patent medicines at a general store or ordered them from mail-order catalogues. Drug distribution was a fairly simple process, largely unregulated by state or federal agencies and affected only by advertising campaigns in magazines and newspapers. American consumers generally got what drugs they wanted, including narcotics, with a modicum of professional intervention by pharmacists. Drug manufacturers produced and promoted their wares without federal interference, relying upon their own internal standards of safety and efficacy. Within a few short decades, however, an increasingly complex network of regulatory standards has governed both the supply of drugs and the professional practice of pharmacy, a phenomenon pharmacy historian Glenn Sonnedecker attributes to inherent safety risks in the supply of drugs, an American trend toward welfare capitalism, and a consumerism movement that "spurs government toward maximizing public safety in all fields, despite economic costs."[5] How did these phenomena affect the American drug distribution system?

By the 1930s, the American health-care system had begun to resemble its current complex configuration. Patients became accustomed to seek professional medical intervention for their serious illnesses, supplemented by visits to the corner drugstore for relief from their minor aches and pains. Sweeping changes in both federal and state laws narrowed the public's access to prescribed drugs while expanding the pharmacist's professional accountability in drug distribution. The nation's pharmaceutical industry, independent from German domination since the end of World War I, began to take on a distinctively American character, aggressively promoting brand-named versions of formulas found in the official compendia. Drugstore chains, once dismissed as nuisances by independent drugstore owners, began to assume a larger, more determined posture in drug distribution, mixing pharmacy practice with variety-store merchandising. A small fraction of pharmacists, disenchanted by the commercialism increasingly associated with retail pharmacy practice, began specializing in providing professional prescription services, including health-related supplies. A new brand of American hospitals, carefully organized for the best service of patients, and emphasizing medical specialties, efficient management, and therapeutic effectiveness, provided the foundation for a more complex system of drug distribution by an emerging new breed of hospital pharmacists.[6]

By mid-century, these trends had become firmly entrenched, increasing the complexity and interdependence that characterized the American drug distribution system. Bolstered by the 1938 Food, Drug and Cosmetic Amendment and the controversial 1951 Durham-Humphrey Amendment, American pharmacists struggled to meet the demands placed upon them by the rapidly expanding medical-care system that emerged in the period of accelerated economic growth following World War II. The American pharmaceutical industry also flourished and consolidated, supplying new and more effective prescription specialties valued at over $1.8 billion by 1958. Physicians relied less upon traditional compounds and prescribed the new, more effective, commercially available drug entities in ever-increasing numbers; indeed, the number of prescriptions dispensed in 1960 had more than quadrupled since 1931.[7] Drugstore chains solidified the gains they had enjoyed since the early 1940s, penetrating and eventually controlling the prescription business they had once abandoned to independent practitioners. Some independent practitioners sought to meet the chains on their own ground, becoming embroiled in ruinous price wars, often forsaking the service ethic that had characterized their practice, while others attempted to emulate Eugene V. White's professional office practice of pharmacy. As the mainstream of medical care shifted from private medical offices and pharmacies into structured, integrated, health-care settings, hospital pharmacists responded to this new environment with enthusiasm and committed themselves to providing pharmaceutical services as an integral part of the total patient-care concept.[8]

## Shifting public perspectives of drug distribution

In recent years, the American drug distribution system has become characterized by even more complex internal and external forces, many of which are no longer under the control of the profession. Internally, pharmaceutical manufacturers, stung by competition from off-patent generic equivalents, produced their own brands of generic products, aggressively sought to shift their safest, most popular prescription drugs to over-the-counter status to increase their market share, and focused their marketing strategies on direct-to-consumer advertising of prescription drugs. In the mid-1990s, aggressive marketing campaigns by major pharmaceutical manufacturers tempted pharmacists into preferred drug product selection with the promise of financial rewards, raising yet another potential for ethical concern.[9] While most drugstore chains consolidated their ranks and began to promote patient-oriented services rather than low prices, deep-discount chains and Internet-based "cyberpharmacies" found their marketing niche among price-conscious consumers who shopped for their prescriptions as they would any other commodity. Beleaguered independent practitioners sought refuge in cooperative buying groups, serviced extended-care facilities, and established specialized practices, focusing upon such areas as durable medical equipment, home-health care, and compounding drugs into unique dosage forms not commercially available. Hospital pharmacists took their expanded clinical services to individual wards, reviewing medication orders, providing pharmacokinetic consults, advising nurses and physicians, taking drug histories from patients, and actively participating in the drug product selection process. Other hospital pharmacists expanded their professional services to the community, competing for the expanding home-health care market created by shorter hospital confinements.

Externally, over the past three decades, governmental agencies, private industry, and university researchers have cooperated in unprecedented ways to improve both the accessibility and availability of health care for the American public. In 1965, for example, the 1935 Social Security Act was amended to create the Medicare and Medicaid programs, which provided access to medical care for older and medically indigent Americans. Within a decade, these regulations were amended again to require pharmacists to perform monthly drug regimen reviews for patients in skilled nursing facilities, and later, to patients in intermediate care facilities. If pharmacists found any problems, they were required to report this information to the medical director. Other federal legislation focussed upon controlling the spiraling cost of health care, instituting a prospective payment system for Medicare patients whereby hospitals were reimbursed on the basis of average hospital confinement costs rather than upon actual costs incurred. These regulations had the effect of releasing patients from hospitals earlier to other facilities (including their homes) where their care could be managed more economically, further stimulating the growth of the home-health care industry. As discussed in Chapter 4, the 1990 Omnibus Budget Reconciliation Act (OBRA) requires health-care providers to furnish written information to their Medicare patients regarding their right to accept or refuse treatment and to formulate instructions explaining how they wish to be treated if they become too ill to express their wishes. Another provision of the Act requires participating states to establish drug utilization review systems, including counseling standards, under which pharmacists must offer to discuss certain matters with their Medicaid patients or their caregivers; many of these enhanced practice standards have been extended to the general public by changes in state pharmacy practice acts or state board regulations. The net effect of the OBRA mandate, according to Abood and Brushwood, "elevates the standard of care owed by pharmacists to all patients."[10]

The foundation for a new American health-care system became more clearly defined during this remarkable period of public policy development. Throughout this process, the issue of prescription drug prices often served as a lightning rod for politicians, consumers, and business executives who wished to control health-care costs. Community and hospital pharmacists alike responded cautiously to the advent of cost-conscious prescription insurance plans and controlled drug formulary programs. By the late 1960s, more than one-third of America's prescription expenditures were covered by so-called "major medical" insurance plans, but only one or two per cent provided prescription coverage on a "first-dollar" basis. By 1974, a third party was paying at least part of the cost of one out of every four prescriptions dispensed in community pharmacies.[11] Community pharmacists were successively annoyed, confused, and nearly overwhelmed by the demands these programs placed upon their practices. Many initially refused to participate in the unstandardized welter of program rules, drug formularies, fee schedules, and claim forms each insurance plan required. Others accepted these burdens and the generally lower dispensing fees and eagerly sought the large-volume prescription business generated by businesses and associations that purchased prescription insurance for their employees. While the introduction of a standardized claim form and computerized data entry systems has softened pharmacists' criticism of these programs, many practitioners feel they have lost both professional and financial control over a significant portion of their practices.

The modern concept of hospital formulary systems is based upon the systematic evaluation and selection of drugs and drug products and established policies of drug use control. Since the 1930s, these systems have drawn upon the strengths of formal liaisons between hospital pharmacists and the medical staff, an arrangement that later became embedded in the Minimum Standard for Hospital Pharmacies of the American College of Surgeons.[12] In recent decades, drug formulary systems have had the practical effect of both limiting the once boundless selection of drug products by physicians while enhancing the influence of hospital pharmacists upon drug product selection in their institutions. Community pharmacists, long accustomed to practicing in an open environment with regard to drug selection, also find themselves constrained by a host of drug formularies established by private insurance companies and government agencies.[13] Obtaining authorization from these companies and agencies to dispense a drug "off the formulary" or from physicians to change their prescribed drug therapy to a product covered under a formulary can pose serious ethical questions for all pharmacy practitioners.

## Impact upon Professional Pharmacy Practice

As we have seen, the expansion of the drug distribution system and the public perspectives of the many rapid changes within that system have created a variety of both professional and ethical challenges to pharmacists, physicians, drug manufacturers, and other members of the health-care community. While these changes have sought to promote efficiency and cost-effectiveness in drug distribution, they have also irrevocably altered time-honored relationships between pharmacists and their patients. Several of these innovations consolidate, fractionate, or otherwise narrow patients' choices of drugs and services, thus minimizing their opportunity to participate in their health-care decision-making. Other innovations, such as direct-to-consumer advertising of prescription drugs or prescription-price advertising, can affect consumer demand for drugs and services, possibly subjecting patients to unnecessary therapy. Still other innovations, such as overly restrictive drug formularies, can deny patients' access to drugs and professional services to which they would otherwise be entitled. Finally, some critics have raised ethical questions about aspects of managed care plans, such as the Coordinated Care Network initially endorsed by the APhA.[14] This Network, which combines the expertise of a major pharmaceutical manufacturer, a national third-party processor, a major mail-order pharmacy service, a national professional pharmacy organization, and thousands of community pharmacies, will attempt to plan and deliver quality pharmaceutical services to specific target audiences.

As the profession of pharmacy enters the twenty-first century, practicing pharmacists will increasingly confront new ethical dilemmas. Among these challenges are the pharmacist's role in assuring fair and equitable prescription pricing, the use of alternative and nontraditional remedies, and the use of narcotics and sedatives to hasten the death of patients for whom life is no longer worth living, an emerging issue that has recently captured the attention of health-system ethicists and practitioners alike.

## Freedom of choice of drugs and services

Pharmacists and physicians have sought efficiency in their professional practices for well over a century. As early as the 1870s, speaking tubes led from fashionable physicians' offices to pharmacists' dispensing areas on a lower floor. Hailed at the time as a quick and efficient method of transmitting prescription orders, the practice was soon criticized as unfair and even unethical (particularly by pharmacists who did not have a tube system) since it necessarily restricted the patient's freedom of choice of pharmacy services. Similar arguments were voiced with the advent of direct telephone lines between physicians' offices and pharmacies, arguments that are echoed today in the controversy over the propriety—and legality—of electronic facsimiles of prescription orders.

One of the most important methods designed to control rising costs in the American health-care system involves the total management of the health-care needs of specific groups of patients by health maintenance organizations (HMOs) and preferred provider organizations (PPOs). Labor unions, teachers' associations, and retiree groups contract with HMOs to provide for their total health-care needs. HMO contracts often require patients to seek their health-care services from a narrowly defined group of providers. Such a "single entry-point" system often includes the provision of pharmacy services, thereby restricting patients' freedom of choice. In contrast, while PPO contracts offer their patients a broader access to services, they are limited to choosing only those providers who agree to the terms of practice specified for the organization.

Today's pharmacists find it increasingly difficult to provide full pharmaceutical care to patients who are also part of a managed care system. Groups of patients may be required to utilize a mail-order prescription service for certain types of medication, particularly maintenance drugs. Patients in these groups are expected to rely upon community pharmacists to compound prescriptions or supply medication for immediate use. This fractionation of pharmacy services can lead to a discontinuity of pharmaceutical care which can be troubling to many pharmacists. The following cases will provide an opportunity to deal with some of these challenges to contemporary pharmacy practice.

## Case 5.1: Directing Prescription Orders

*"I just got your fax prescription from Dr. Bell, Mrs. Dare."*

Dr. Bell has just completed his annual routine physical of Mrs. Ginny Dare. "Everything seems to be in order, Mrs. Dare," Dr. Bell assures her. "I would like to change the strength of your estrogen therapy, however. I'll just fax this prescription to the pharmacist downstairs." Mrs. Dare is a little puzzled because she always has her prescriptions filled at her neighborhood pharmacy, but does not question Dr. Bell about the matter, assuming she will be able to pick up the prescription order downstairs. Pharmacist Chuck Tufts greets Mrs. Dare warmly. "I just got your prescription from Dr. Bell, Mrs. Dare. I'll have it ready for you in a few minutes." "No, no, young man!" Mrs. Dare exclaims. "I want to take my prescription to the pharmacy near my home." Chuck has never released a faxed prescription to a patient before, although such prescriptions are legal in his state. What is Chuck's obligation to Mrs. Dare? What important underlying moral principles govern this situation?

**Commentary:** The 1848 Code of Ethics of the Philadelphia College of Pharmacy declared as unjust to the profession and injurious to the public any pharmacist's act that allowed physicians a percentage of or commission on prescriptions being compounded and dispensed. Such an attitude about unethical "monied interest" persisted between America's physicians and pharmacists, albeit in varying forms, throughout the twentieth century. More recently, with the advent of rigidly structured medical service systems like HMOs and PPOs, the practice linkage between pharmacists and physicians has expanded into more complex alliances, often for the betterment of the patient, but are still subject to critique and question. This case illustrates a simple closed linkage where the prescribing physician employs a facsimile ("fax") system, allowing the linked pharmacist to directly capture the drug request. Pharmacist Chuck Tufts has a range of options open to him. Assuming that the linkage between Chuck and Dr. Bell is above reproach and done solely with a view toward improving service to patients, any "kickback" criticism can be ignored and only those options dealing with the remaining moral issues considered. If Chuck were ruled only by doing "what's good for the patient," he could insist on filling the prescription for Mrs. Dare; if she refuses, then she will not get any medicine. There are obvious and forbidding prohibitions for choosing this action. Denying service to any patient in order to serve the system would be judged wrong by any internal or external standard of professional behavior. Chuck could also provide a copy of the facsimile prescription to Mrs. Dare without further comment, allowing her to have it filled elsewhere. This would respect some of Mrs. Dare's rights as a patient, but unless Chuck discusses the fax system and the importance of the planned linkage with Mrs. Dare and Dr. Bell's need to monitor her therapy, this option has little to recommend itself. Finally, Chuck could provide full and understandable disclosure about the linked physician-pharmacist arrangement to Mrs. Dare, along with complete and amiable discussion with the ultimate dispensing pharmacist. In this manner, Chuck will be respecting not only the rights of the patient but also the relationship between Mrs. Dare and her chosen pharmacist.

### Case 5.2: Limiting Access to Service

*"Sorry, I can't fill your HMO prescriptions."*

"Rufe" Rorem is a 55-year-old steelworker employed by a local mill. His union recently contracted with Total Health Care, Inc., a single entry-point HMO. Rufe has sustained numerous injuries over the years and has been a loyal patron of Lloyd's Pharmacy for many years. Jack Lloyd maintains scrupulous prescription profiles and takes pride in providing the highest standard of pharmacy care. Rufe is often a little confused, and sometimes can be difficult to deal with. Today, Rufe brings in a prescription from a physician employed by his new HMO. "I hope you have this stuff, Jack," Rufe drawls, "my leg is hurtin' somethin' fierce." Jack glances at the prescription for a new nonsteroidal antiinflammatory that is notorious for causing serious drug interactions, particularly in patients such as Rufe. He recalls that the pharmacy services included in Rufe's new HMO contract must be obtained directly from the HMO pharmacy. Jack regrets that he will no longer be able to provide the full continuity of pharmacy care that he knows Rufe needs, but feels he has no choice. He tries to explain his dilemma to an increasingly irritated and confused Rufe. "Sorry, I can't fill your HMO prescriptions," Jack concludes somewhat lamely. "I hope you understand." Rufe limps away muttering under his breath. What moral dilemma does Jack face? Does Jack have a moral duty to assure that Rufe obtains his medication? How would a virtue-centered ethic assist Jack in this situation?

**Commentary:** One of the principles of the 1994 Code of Ethics for Pharmacists heralds the integrity of pharmacists in professional relationships and their pledge to be truthful and act with the conviction of their conscience. Pharmacists, like all members of moral communities, claim the right to professional autonomy and thus reserve the right to make decisions based on values, standards, and preferences established by the profession itself. Consequently, the right to refuse to fill a prescription order, although not an absolute right, stands as a foundational prerogative of professional pharmacy practice. In this case, Jack Lloyd has decided to refuse Rufe his needed antiinflammatory medicine, thereby causing at least some level of consternation. This would seem to be a defensible action since Jack is attempting to prevent possible harm to Rufe, yet it leaves Rufe in a quandary, perhaps confused about what to do next. Jack could counsel Rufe about the use of the intended medication, including his concerns about potential drug interactions, allowing Rufe to participate in deciding whether or not the medication should be used. In this case, Jack would be demonstrating his respect for Rufe's right of self-determination as well as protecting Rufe's right to have the drug product prescribed by his physician. Furthermore, Jack will need to guard against possible complications, such as Rufe's concerns about not having received this kind of information from his physician or explaining to Rufe in greater detail the need to have this type of prescription filled within the coordinated HMO system.

### Case 5.3: Fractionating Pharmacy Services

*"I just need a few pills until my mail order comes."*

Professor Rowland Hill enters Alexander's Pharmacy with two new prescriptions in his hand. "Good morning, Mr. Alexander," Professor Hill says brightly. "I'd like these filled, please." Maury Alexander studies the two prescriptions. One is for a ten-day supply of a powerful antibiotic, the other is for a week's supply of hydrochlorothiazide, a drug Maury knows Professor Hill has been taking for several years. "I have a deep puncture wound in my foot," Professor Hill explains ruefully. "My doctor wanted me to start that antibiotic immediately." Maury is a little puzzled. "Is your doctor reevaluating your blood-pressure medication?" "Oh, no," Professor Hill replies, "I just need a few pills until my mail order comes." Professor Hill has been a patient of Maury's for several years, and he is troubled by this new development. First, he feels he will not be able to completely monitor Professor Hill's drug use if some of his medications are supplied from another source. Secondly, he knows Professor Hill will object to the prescription fee he must charge for seven tablets of hydrochlorothiazide. Finally, he feels somehow "used" by the system of managed care Professor Hill's group has chosen to provide pharmacy services, and feel tempted to refuse to fill either prescription. Why is Maury so troubled? Does his conflict stem from a virtue-centered ethic or some other source? What should Maury do?

Commentary: Maintaining patients' freedom to select their attending health-care professionals continues to evolve as a contentious issue in contemporary medical practice. When nearly all medical and drug charges were on a fee-for-service basis and paid for privately, patients exercised their right to choose their physician and pharmacist. Today, the availability of professional services has become much more complex and restrictive, making this relished "freedom of choice" less absolute. This case places the freedom of choice claimed by the patient into conflict with patient-care management. Maury Alexander is facing a common practice dilemma, providing professional services to a patient whose medication regimen is complicated by having multiple sources for his pharmacy services. Maury is asked to provide the antibiotic Professor Hill needs as well as a few diuretic tablets to hold him over until he receives his full diuretic prescription from an alternate source. Apparently troubled by both ethical and clinical concerns, Maury ponders the advisability of denying services to Professor Hill as a possible solution. He believes he is justified in taking this action because of this concern for Professor Hill's well-being, but also by the likelihood of being viewed by Professor Hill as being unfair in charging so much for a few "water pills." Maury's feeling of estrangement caused by an intrusive outside system strongly supports this alternative, yet Maury is disturbed by the thought of denying services to Professor Hill and wonders if such an act is truly warranted. Maury needs to extend his deliberations beyond his somewhat self-serving conclusions that he is outside the patient-care loop, liable to be viewed by Professor Hill as unfair in his prescription pricing, and generally being "used" by the system. If

Maury is truthful to his relationship with Professor Hill, he will need to devise a course of action that moves beyond the self-serving denial of services.

## The fully informed consumer of drugs and services

Just as patients rely upon their physicians to fully inform them of both the intended benefits and the possible risks of any proposed therapy or procedure, consumers also rely upon their pharmacists to provide enough truthful information to allow them to make informed choices about prescription drugs and services. As noted in Chapter 4, one of the most contentious ethical issues in recent years focussed upon the advertising of prescription prices and services. Consumers argued they had a right to learn about prescription prices and services through advertising, enabling them to shop wisely; pharmacists countered that the practice promoted unfair competition and was inherently unethical. Since the mid-1970s, changing ethical standards and a new openness in dealing with patients has quelled that debate, yet the advertising of prices alone can still be misleading and can undermine patients' judgment, distorting their ability to make an informed choice.

Patients also expect their pharmacists to provide truthful information about the prescription drugs they dispense. Since the advent of generic drugs and multisourced pharmaceuticals and the repeal of the so-called "antisubstitution laws" across the nation, consumers have been asked to choose between a branded pharmaceutical or its generic counterpart, often on the basis of little or no factual information. Pharmacists have struggled trying to convey the concept of generic equivalency to their patients, only to be asked which drug is cheaper. Too often patients make uninformed choices of their drug products on the basis of price alone. By condoning such uninformed choices, pharmacists contribute to a diminished standard of pharmaceutical care.

Finally, direct-to-consumer advertising of prescription drugs in the print and electronic media poses a potential ethical challenge to physicians and pharmacists alike. While such advertising is not inherently unethical, many question if it is appropriate to advertise potentially dangerous drugs in this manner or if sufficient information can be conveyed through these ads to permit consumers to make an informed self-diagnosis. Physicians argue that such advertising creates a demand for a drug for which there may be no real medical need and may even contribute to drug abuse. Pharmacists argue that direct-to-consumer prescription drug advertising interferes with or even undermines the physician-patient-pharmacist relationship. The following cases provide practice in examining these issues.

### Case 5.4: Advertising Prescription Prices

*"$5 OFF ANY NEW Rx WITH THIS COUPON!"*

An excited Rex Tugwell entered Painter's Pharmacy waving a small piece of paper in his hand. "Look at this coupon, Doc!" he exclaimed. "The new drugstore down the street is really wheeling and dealing." Lynn Painter sighed. He had already endured several similar encounters with other patients earlier in the day. Lynn patiently explained that he was not able or willing to meet the competition on this promotion, pointing out that the new pharmacy did not offer the full range of professional services that his pharmacy did. Rex was not impressed with Lynn's response. "I figure you guys are overcharging me by at least five bucks anyway," he retorted. "Why don't you just forget the gimmicks and charge us fair prescription prices to start with." Lynn realizes that Rex is uninformed and confused about this issue. How should he respond? What ethical dilemma does this case illustrate? What ethical principles could Lynn examine to help him resolve this problem?

**Commentary:** The question of price competition among pharmacies has been an ethical concern in professional pharmacy practice for over 150 years. The 1848 Code of Ethics of the Philadelphia College of Pharmacy warned of the injury caused by this sort of behavior and cautioned that "no apothecary should intentionally undersell his neighbors." The 1852 APhA Code of Ethics also cautioned against intentional reductions in the rate of charges among apothecaries believing such action to be "productive of evil results." Eventually, these principles evolved into less proscriptive statements, urging pharmacists to receive only "fair and honest remuneration for their professional services." The 1994 Code of Ethics for Pharmacists relies entirely on the virtues of honesty and integrity for guidance in this matter. As this case demonstrates, the clash between the "business" and the "professional" sides of pharmacy practice will always be difficult. Pharmacist Lynn Painter has at least two options open to him: He can tell Rex to take advantage of the best deal available to him or he can provide Rex the kind of information that he will need to become a more informed consumer of health-care services. In either case, Lynn will need to be cautious, attempting to balance his commitment toward honesty and integrity with respect toward his colleagues.

### Case 5.5: Choosing among Multisource Drugs

*"I'd like to use this other brand in your prescription."*

Pharmacist Alice Halstead is upset. Ray Wilbur has just handed her a prescription from Dr. Christie for an expensive brand of a cephalosporin which is available from other manufacturers at a greatly reduced price. Dr. Christie is a cantankerous elderly practitioner who unsuccessfully fought the repeal of the state antisubstitution law several years ago and takes out his frustration by writing "DAW" on all his prescriptions. Alice knows that the more expensive brand Dr. Christie prescribed for Mr. Wilbur has no real therapeutic advantage over the less expensive brands and decides to ignore Dr. Christie's direction and dispense a less expensive brand, one in which she has full confidence. Alice explains the DAW rule to Mr. Wilbur and her rationale for wishing to dispense an alternate brand. "I'd like to use this other brand in your prescription, Mr. Wilbur," Alice concludes. "What do you think?" Mr. Wilbur enthusiastically supports Alice's therapeutic plan, and adds, "Why, this is wonderful, Alice. I'll be sure to mention this to Dr. Christie the next time I see him." Is Alice justified in ignoring Dr. Christie's directive? Should Mr. Wilbur's intended disclosure to Dr. Christie affect Alice's decision?

**Commentary:** Pharmacists and all members of the health-care professions have a stake in helping consumers of drugs and professional services become fully informed, attesting to their moral obligation to respect patients' rights to autonomy and foster their right of self-determination. In developing a foundation for attaining this level of patient care, pharmacists often encounter issues that appear peripheral to a physician's therapeutic intent, such as the availability of lower cost but therapeutically equivalent drug products or seemingly irresponsible restraints placed upon the dispensing process by prescribing physicians or state pharmacy practice acts. Nevertheless, these side issues can significantly affect the intensity and extent of patient communication that contributes to creating a truly informed patient. Alice Halstead has several options available to her, all depending upon how she responds to several important initial questions. Since Dr. Christie wrote "DAW" on his prescription, the state pharmacy practice act requires Alice to dispense the exact drug product Dr. Christie has prescribed. By contravening this law, Alice may feel her value position—using lower-cost drug products—is more valid than Dr. Christie's unreasonable insistence that all his prescription must be filled as written. Although Alice included Mr. Wilbur in her decision process, she excludes Dr. Christie, possibly wishing to avoid a disagreeable and unproductive confrontation. Alice could decide not to dispense the prescription and return it to Mr. Wilbur on the grounds of not agreeing with the practice option of Dr. Christie. Denying professional service is a drastic option, but Alice could defend it based upon what she believes is in the best interest of the patient, a lower-cost, therapeutically equivalent drug product. Unfortunately, this would not help Mr. Wilbur's medical problem and might cause it to worsen. Suppose Mr. Wilbur is elderly, has no immediate transportation to the next available pharmacy, and agrees to the cost of the more expensive product. Would this be enough for Alice to relent?

### Case 5.6: Direct-to-Consumer Advertising

*"Doc, I saw this ad on TV last night . . ."*

Pharmacist Fred Taylor is sipping his third cup of coffee one morning when the telephone rings. Fred recognizes the distinctive nasal twang of "Phi" Farnsworth, one of Fred's steady customers. "Doc, I saw this ad on TV last night about a new drug for hay fever and it sounds great." Fred rolls his eyes as he listens to Mr. Farnsworth describe a new prescription-only antihistamine that has recently been heavily advertised to the public on television and the print media. Fred is concerned about these new direct-to-consumer promotions because he feels that the ads do not provide the public with enough information. Mr. Farnsworth asks Fred to telephone his physician to get a prescription for the new drug. Fred knows that Mr. Farnsworth is already maintained on adequate antihistamine therapy, but realizes that his physician will probably go along with any recommendation Fred might make in this matter. What is the ethical issue in this case? Does Fred have an ethical obligation to inform Mr. Farnsworth about his concerns?

**Commentary:** Promoting the use of nonprescription drug products directly to the consumer has been an important segment of the marketing practices of the American pharmaceutical industry for more than a century. This practice has fostered and nourished the American fascination with self-medication that is supported by these products. In the last decade, the industry has developed a direct-to-consumer (DTC) promotion of prescription drug products as part of its marketing strategy, causing some concerns among pharmacists and other health-care professionals. Supposedly, the basis for DTC promotion is to heighten the interest and increase the knowledge level of potential consumers of these prescription drug products. Armed with this information, these consumers would contact their prescribing physicians and inquire about the availability and possible use of these products to treat their often self-diagnosed medical conditions. The ethical issues surrounding DTC practices may not be apparent. Certainly, if the drug product being promoted carries with it genuine benefits for the patient, either as a new treatment or as an improvement on an existing treatment at no greater cost, there would seem to be no reason to suspect an ethical challenge. Drug products that provide identical treatment at a substantially lower cost may be reasonable candidates for DTC promotion. Using DTC techniques to promote products simply to capture or increase market share may not be unethical, but hovers close to the questionable level. On the surface, providing legitimate drug product information to the general public does not appear to contravene any moral principle. DTC strategies may even seem laudable since they freely make available the kind of information that is needed for a fully informed consumer. However, in examining DTC promotions for the presence of ethical dilemmas it may be necessary to move beyond the mere promotional material and scrutinize underlying factors. Why is the producer of the product going directly to the consumers? Is the material presented understandable by a majority of interested potential patients or only those with a sophisticated medical background? Is DTC being used to circumvent the screening effect of prescribing physicians or does it put pressure on those physicians who are reluctant to try something new? Are patients being targeted unfairly, playing on their fears of medical intervention? Fred Taylor has encountered a DTC situation with a twist: His patient, Phi Farnsworth, has asked him to intervene on his behalf with his physician. Phi has heard of a new, possibly better drug product and wants his doctor to prescribe it for his use. Fred has a major role to play in this situation, starting with a full examination of the purposes and intent of the DTC promotion. In addition, he will need to decide exactly what kind of information he needs to discuss with Phi. It may not be possible for Fred to explain DTC to Phi and any potential ethical dilemmas he sees without causing Phi some distress.

## Access to drugs and professional services

Pharmacists have traditionally served as protectors of the public health by scrupulously guarding the public's access to potentially dangerous drugs and devices. In recent years, this important professional function has assumed greater importance, particularly with regard to professional services, a function that carries with it expanded ethical responsibilities. While very few, if any, pharmacists would deny professional services to patients based on their race, cultural background, or personal appearance, many find that they are increasingly forced to deny professional services to some patients due to constraining policies established by state pharmacy practice acts, governmental reimbursement programs, insurance carriers, and medical researchers. These policies can create ethical dilemmas for the pharmacist, as the following cases illustrate.

### Case 5.7: Exercising Professional Discretion

*"Do you carry any quinine capsules?"*

Sixteen-year-old Marie Stopes enters Finlay Pharmacy with a worried look on her face. "Good morning, Mr. Finlay," she says quietly. "Do you carry any quinine capsules?" "Why, yes, Marie," Alex Finlay smiles. "We carry both the three- and five-grain capsules, and they don't require a prescription." "That's great," Marie replies. "I'd like a dozen of the five-grain capsules, please." Marie continues to chat with Alex as he prepares her order. "I understand you are supposed to take two capsules every four hours. Is that right?" Alex looks over his glasses at her. "That's a rather high dose, Marie," he replies cautiously. "Are you experiencing cramps?" "No," Marie replies quietly, avoiding his gaze. "I just need it for something else, that's all." Alex realizes that Marie is probably purchasing the quinine capsules to induce an abortion. What is his ethical responsibility in this situation? Is Marie's age a factor in this case? Is Alex justified in seeking more information? Upon what ethical grounds might he refuse to supply the capsules to Marie?

**Commentary:** The Hippocratic Oath, often cited by the general public as the ultimate code of ethics for physicians, clearly warns against the distribution of any "abortive remedy." No such prohibition has ever been expressed in pharmacy's codes of ethics, although the public and pharmacists alike assume that the distribution of nonprescription abortive remedies would not be acceptable in professional pharmacy practice. Over the years, however, many anecdotal stories have emerged about pharmacists who provide such products as quinine, slippery elm bark, and Humphrey's No. 11 Homeopathic Remedy to the public, all purported abortive remedies. Neither the 2001 Principles of Medical Ethics of the American Medical Association nor the 1994 Code of Ethics for Pharmacists include any reference to abortifacients, relying solely upon the patient-medical practitioner relationship as guidance for their members. In this case, Alex Finlay faces a complex situation involving a 16-year-old girl who might be seeking an abortive remedy, although he does not have any confirmation that Marie will actually be using the quinine capsules for this purpose. Alex faces a number of issues that further contribute to this dilemma, including, perhaps, personally held values that could prohibit him from engaging in any activity linked with abortion. Of equal concern to Alex may be the nature of the professional relationship that exists between himself and Marie, especially since Alex believes there is additional information he needs from Marie. At best, Alex will have to balance a response that lies between his belief in what may be an immoral act and the need to prevent a patient from potential harm. Distraught and cautious, Marie is not being completely forthright in her dealings with Alex; nevertheless, she is seeking assistance in what she considers to be a critical moment in her life. If Alex considers his personally held stance on abortion to be defensible and compelling, he needs to fully disclose this attitude to Marie and caution her against proceeding with the venture. Furthermore, if Marie is pregnant and seeking care and comfort, Alex will need to examine an array of reasonable support sources for her to consider. Alex might also accept the notion that because the facts of the situation are insufficient and further information not forthcoming, he will need to act on the matter as it exists. Marie is entitled to not only professional pharmacy services that are based on her needs and the information provided, but also to be treated with full respect for her autonomy. Alex needs to provide the consequences of high-dosage quinine therapy as objectively as possible, especially with regard to its toxicity and untoward reactions, and rely upon Marie's self-determination.

### Case 5.8: Managing Third-Party Program Conflicts

*"I'm sorry, Doctor, that drug isn't covered."*

The telephone interrupts Joe Remington's Medicaid billing routine. "Good morning, Joe," Dr. Gregory says briskly. "I'd like Roby Kaye to have four ounces of Robitussin AC, one teaspoonful q4h." Joe has just entered a Medicaid claim for Roby and knows that over-the-counter drugs are not covered by the state Medicaid program. "I'm sorry, Doctor, that drug isn't covered by Medicaid," Joe replies tactfully. "Would you consider . . ." "Joe," Dr. Gregory interrupts brusquely, "I refuse to change my prescribing habits because of those damn Medicaid regs. Just do as I ask." Roby shuffles slowly into Joe's pharmacy. "Mornin', Mr. Remington," Roby wheezes. "Do you have my cough syrup ready?" Joe faces a real dilemma. He realizes that he could fill the prescription as written and bill Medicaid for an another drug that is covered, an alternative he knows constitutes fraud. He also knows that Roby cannot pay for the over-the-counter cough syrup himself, and would probably refuse treatment. Should Joe bring Roby into his decision-making process? How does Joe balance his duty to Roby with his obligations to the law and to society? What ethical principles apply in this case?

**Commentary:** The conflict that is often felt by members of moral communities as they endeavor to observe the rules of law while engaging in their professional practices manifests itself in many forms. Until recently, codes of ethics within the profession of pharmacy have warned pharmacists of their obligation to observe the law and not engage in any activity that will bring discredit to the profession. As the health-care delivery system continues to increase in complexity, especially with the additional constraints of cost-control measures such as closed formularies, practice conflicts that test pharmacists' determination to observe rules of law are not only increasing in frequency, but are also becoming more varied in nature. These practice conflicts are particularly trying for pharmacists as they attempt to more fully implement the practice philosophy of pharmaceutical care and respond to the aspirations of the

1994 Code of Ethics for Pharmacists. Meeting the needs of patients with care and compassion in the light of these confounding legal restraints may require practice attitudes and responses that are far beyond ordinary and casual professional practice procedures. Joe Remington is faced with the challenge of how to provide the needed drug therapy to Roby and remain within the legal bounds of the Medicaid system. Because of Dr. Gregory's adamant attitude, Joe is stymied in his attempt to dispense an alternate legend drug to Roby and begins to rationalize an action that will provide an over-the-counter product to Roby, but which will also involve a fraudulent billing process. Such an action seems attractive, since both Roby and Dr. Gregory will be served and Joe will be reimbursed for his service. Unfortunately, the solution violates the Medicaid laws, and while Joe is at risk of being prosecuted for fraud, he believes his illegal act is more acceptable than any other action that would be harmful to Roby. It would be unfortunate if Joe does not consider other courses of action he might follow in solving this practice challenge. For example, Joe might pursue a candid discussion with Roby, carefully explaining not only the formulation of Robitussin AC, but also the fundamentals of prescription versus nonprescription designations for drug products, leading, perhaps, to a resolution that would be prompted by Roby himself. This might be the most desirable approach, since the only problem Joe would have is one of reimbursement for his services; there are no questions either about Roby's need for the drug or its efficacy. Other resolutions are obvious, some of which are undesirable: Joe could decide the aggravation of dealing with Dr. Gregory and rigid third-party programs is too great, and he could squirm away from the problem by telling Roby that he doesn't have the product, thus solving his problem but not really helping Roby. He might consider offering to sell Roby the product as an over-the-counter drug, perhaps in its generic form at a greatly reduced cost. Finally, Joe might consider the product as a prescription, provide Roby full counseling, extend credit for a non-Medicaid prescription charge, and take his chances on future reimbursement. Regardless of which approach Joe decides upon, he ought to include Roby in all aspects of the decision-making process. Ultimately, Joe's choice will be a reflection of his devotion to virtue-based ethics and whether generosity and altruism are also included in his vision of treating patients with care and compassion.

## Case 5.9: Participating in Investigational Studies

*"Tell me what the doctor told you about your new drug."*

Sue Hayhurst is a clinical pharmacist in a large university-based research hospital. One of her responsibilities entails taking drug histories of all patients engaged in investigational studies of new drugs and providing counseling to patients concerning these drugs. Ed Dodds has been selected for participation in a new study involving an investigational drug for prostate cancer. Sue enters Mr. Dodds's room and introduces herself to him. Mr. Dodds is an elderly, outgoing man with a florid face. Sue begins her counseling, but soon realizes that Mr. Dodds seems to be quite vague about his participation in the study. "Tell me what the doctor told you about your new drug," Sue asks. "Well, he didn't say much of anything, Miss," Mr. Dodds replies with a chuckle. "He just had me sign some papers and left." Sue realizes that Mr. Dodds has no idea of the risks associated with the experimental therapy and that his signed informed consent form is essentially meaningless. What is Sue's duty to Mr. Dodds? Should she discuss her concerns with Mr. Dodds at this point or consult with his physician first? What should Sue do if his physician refuses to take corrective measures?

Commentary: The use of informed consent procedures, introduced in the mid-twentieth century as a manifestation of the respect for the autonomous person, is a relatively new practice concept in medicine. It may be the most important practice available for safeguarding against the abuse of human subjects in investigational studies of new drugs. Pharmacists who understand the issues underlying the ethical principle of respect for autonomy and the concept of informed consent are better equipped to understand the ethical issues that confront investigational drug research. The most common form of informed consent consists of a legal document that explains the risks and benefits of a procedure or research study and which is signed by the research subjects as evidence of their consent. Ethicists argue that morally valid informed consent requires both a written assent form and a conversation with the subject patient. Furthermore, the disclosure must be sufficient and understandable and the patient needs to be competent and free to act without being compelled in any way. Such communication elements provide the basis for making informed consent in a true au-

tonomous function, not as a mere function of policy. Sue Hayhurst
has apparently concluded that Mr. Dodds has not been adequately
informed about the investigational drug therapy and therefore has
not provided valid informed consent. Fortunately, Sue has encountered this dilemma at the onset of the investigation; had she discovered the predicament during actual drug dosing, she would be
faced with a weightier moral dilemma, the withholding of a potentially beneficial drug treatment. Sue's duty in this case is fairly
clear: If she believes, as a member of pharmacy's moral community,
that her services are based on professional autonomy, then she
needs to respect Mr. Dodds's autonomy. Mr. Dodds has clearly indicated through his fragmented and partial responses, that he is either not competent enough to provide consent to this research procedure or was not provided the information necessary to make an
informed decision. How Sue proceeds to assure Mr. Dodds's right of
self-determination presents her with potentially serious challenges.
The 1994 Code of Ethics for Pharmacists affirms both the
pharmacist's respect for the values and abilities of health-care colleagues and the duty to act with honesty and integrity in professional relations. In light of these principles, Sue ought to have a
private conversation with the physician in charge of the research
project and attempt to confirm her conclusions concerning the validity of Mr. Dodds's informed consent. Mr. Dodds's responses to
her questions may be characteristic of some long-standing physical
malady well-known to the attending physician and the actual informed consent obtained orally through an acceptable surrogate,
perhaps Mrs. Dodds. If this is not the case and Sue maintains her
objection to the validity of Mr. Dodds's assent, she will need to
convince the research director of her finding and seek further resolution. Sue may also feel she needs to inform Mr. Dodds of her concerns and how she is attempting to correct them, especially if the
physician in charge of the project politely rebuffs Sue's claim of infringement and continues the investigation. Sue also might wish to
meet with the medical center's institutional review board for a
complete review of her concerns and determine their course of action at the institutional level.

## Dealing with terminal illness

As the post-World War II "baby boomers" begin to age and become infirm, many are faced with difficult decisions concerning the
declining quality of their lives; some are forced to consider whether
or not they should take measures to end their lives. Modern medi-

cal science is a two-edged sword: On one hand, we have developed drugs and medical procedures that can prolong life almost indefinitely; on the other hand, we have an increasing population of older Americans for whom life is no longer worth living. Some senior citizens feel compelled to spend down their life savings to extend the life of a loved one in a coma for a few precious weeks. Indeed, it is estimated that nearly 80 per cent of a person's lifelong health-care costs are spent during the last few weeks of life. While many would recoil at the term "euthanasia," there is a growing body of literature that supports a person's right to die.

When faced with refractory symptoms that cannot be controlled without the patient losing consciousness, physicians have few alternatives open to them. Under certain rigid circumstances, the physician must judge that palliative care is unlikely to provide adequate relief to the terminally ill patient within a tolerable period of time. In consultation with the patient and his or her caregivers, the physician may choose among three options: providing a lethal dose of a drug that the patient takes voluntarily (physician-assisted suicide), administering a lethal dose to a patient who may no longer be able to care for his or her personal needs (active voluntary euthanasia), or employing high—but not lethal—doses of drugs that induce a deep sleep (terminal sedation). In cases of terminal sedation, physicians and pharmacists monitor terminally ill patients over a period of several days or weeks, adjusting dosages to ensure that the patients are not suffering. Eventually, these patients pass away in their sleep. While purists would argue that the difference between managing the death of a patient with drugs and euthanasia is a distinction without a difference, the practice of terminal sedation is growing. What is the pharmacist's ethical responsibilities in such cases? Some pharmacists' personal belief systems cannot accommodate the termination of life under any circumstances; these pharmacists would be advised to refer these special patients to another pharmacist. For those who find these issues troubling, the following cases may prove illuminating:

### Case 5.10: Managing Cases of Terminal Sedation

*"Doctor, I'm troubled by this prescription."*

Pharmacist Ed Patch has a problem. He has just received a prescription for an unusually strong dose of a sedative for Mr. Durkheim, one of his long-time patients who has recently been confined to bed for a terminal illness. In checking the prescription order with Dr. Menninger, he is surprised to learn that the dosage schedule is correct and that Mr. Durkheim and his family have agreed to discontinue further treatment, including nutrition and hydration, totally sedate Mr. Durkheim, and allow him to pass away quietly in his sleep. Ed has always held the health and well-being of his patients as his highest concern, and he is disturbed that one of his patients has entered into such an agreement to end his own life. Ed's discussion with Dr. Menninger has confirmed that Mr. Durkheim faces a long and painful ordeal that could last for several weeks. Ed is reluctant to fill the prescription, but realizes that Mr. Durkheim would continue to experience a long and painful period of decline before his death. What should Ed do? Are there any provisions in the 1994 Code of Ethics for Pharmacists that Ed can look to for guidance?

**Commentary:** Situations such as the one that pharmacist Ed Patch has encountered are now a reality of professional pharmacy practice, so much so that the phrases "pharmaceutically mediated death" and "pharmaceutically assisted death" have been added to the medical lexicon. These enigmatic phrases embody a range of clinical activities, including terminal sedation, and are important to profession of pharmacy because they highlight the role pharmacists play in these cases. Moreover, these phrases underscore the importance of decisions made by pharmacists as they struggle to meet their obligations in providing quality pharmaceutical care. Indeed, some authors argue that the failure of effective pharmaceutical care is a necessary condition for pharmaceutically mediated death.[15] There is no universally accepted definition of terminal sedation; however, most clinicians describe the effort as: 1) intentionally producing and maintaining deep sleep, but not deliberately causing death, and 2) entering into an agreement with the patient stating that when the patient reaches a point at which his or her condition is intractable or refractory to standard palliative treatment and is in a deep sleep, the patient will no longer receive any further supportive treatment, allowing death to occur. Some clinicians prefer to name this procedure "palliative sedation" or "sedation in the imminently dying."[16]

This case presents challenges on many fronts. Traditionally, pharmacists have recognized a moral, even legal, duty to fill valid prescriptions; at present, some pharmacists question their right of refusal to fill prescriptions on the grounds of conscience. Ed will first have to settle that issue and in so doing will need to more completely examine the circumstances of the case. Ed will need to ascertain the intention of the physician in proposing terminal sedation; he also will need to be satisfied that the explicit intention of the prescribed sedative is for the relief of suffering and not the hastening of death. Furthermore, Ed will need to confirm that the patient made a voluntary and informed choice for sedation and refusal of food and fluids. Once these facts are confirmed, Ed can decide whether or not he wants to cooperate by preparing the medication. In making his decision, Ed will probably be torn between two widely held principles of moral behavior: the avoidance of killing and autonomy.

Although the principle of avoidance of killing is not specifically addressed in the Code of Ethics for Pharmacists, it seems apparent to Ed that killing is just inherently wrong, even if the patients who die are better off than if they had lived. While Dr. Menninger has assured Ed that the intent of the sedative was not the death of the Mr. Durkheim, Ed realizes what the ultimate outcome will be. At the same time, Ed recognizes and fully supports the respect for patient autonomy statement in the Code of Ethics for Pharmacists, and concludes that Mr. Durkheim has the right to decide such an outcome for himself. In order to resolve this matter, Ed will need to carefully examine these principles and decide if one principle has priority over the other, whether the principles need to be balanced against each other, or whether they can be combined for a final resolution to the challenge.

### Case 5.11: Managing Cases of Euthanasia

*"We have no other recourse for Mr. Gehrig"*

Pharmacist Bill Simpson gulps a quick cup of coffee on his way to the meeting of the Critical Care Committee. The Committee has been wrestling with some difficult issues of late, most involving terminally ill patients. Dr. Charcot presents a case that immediately grabs Bill's attention. Mr. Gehrig, who suffers from amyotrophic lateral sclerosis, is no longer able to feed himself and finds life to be unbearable. He begs Dr. Charcot to provide him with enough sedatives to end his misery; his family supports his decision. While hospital policy does not allow such interventions, Dr. Charcot convinces the Committee that administrating a large dose under such circumstances is an acceptable treatment plan. "We have

no other recourse for Mr. Gehrig," he concludes. Bill is uncomfortable dispensing such a large dose to Mr. Gehrig because he
knows that he will undoubtedly die. Can Bill refuse to fill the
prescription order? What justification could Jack use to
change Dr. Charcot's treatment plan?

**Commentary:** In recent years, the role of health professionals
in assisting patients in bringing about their deaths has become a
major medical, social, and political issue. In the Netherlands, physicians may perform euthanasia upon the persistent request of the
patient; here in the United States, the state of Oregon has its
Death with Dignity Act that allows for physician-assisted suicide
where the patient consumes a lethal dose of a drug, a dose dispensed by a consenting pharmacist. Both of these systems carefully restrict euthanasia to patients who have made a voluntary request while they were mentally competent and able to make
substantially autonomous choices. Nevertheless, when a competent
patient experiences profound and genuinely intractable suffering
and makes a fully informed and voluntary request for lethal assistance, the health professional will need to decide whether voluntary
choice can justify mercy killings.

In this case, Dr. Charcot asks pharmacist Bill Simpson to cooperate in the killing of Mr. Gehrig by preparing the medication. Even
if Bill agrees that Mr. Gehrig has the right to kill himself, he may be
unsure whether he has the moral right to assist in the procedure by
preparing a lethal dose of the medication and thereby assist in his
death. Some members of society might argue that mercy killing and
assisted-suicide are defensible; however, most health practitioners
maintain there is something incompatible between their role as
health-care professionals and these acts. Bill has no difficulty in complying with treatment plans that use medications to make the patient
more comfortable while they die, even if the medications hasten their
death as a side effect, but here the direct outcome intended is the
death of Mr. Gehrig. Bill faces the tension between avoiding killing
and maintaining respect for Mr. Gehrig's autonomy.

## Controlling the prices of prescription medication

Prior to the 1940s, it was not unusual for a pharmacist to compound a dozen prescriptions during a day's work for not much more
than a dozen dollars. Pharmacists often extended credit to their
patients during the Great Depression, sometimes even providing

indigent patients with drugs at no charge. With the advent of brand-name drugs in the 1950s, prescription drug prices increased modestly, prompting congressional investigations and the subsequent introduction of generic equivalents. By the 1990s, with the introduction of more potent, specific drug products which were now advertised directly to the public, drug prices soared. Even pharmacists who wished to provide *pro bono* services to the indigent could no longer afford to do so; others were limited by corporate policy. To some, it seemed that the American free-enterprise system of pharmaceutical research and development was out of control. The pharmaceutical industry defended its pricing schedules by self-righteously pointing to the escalating costs of developing new drug products and the cost of marketing these new products over a foreshortened period of patent protection. The average citizen, responding to rapidly rising prescription prices, was unconvinced. Citizen action groups called upon the federal government to launch further investigations; the pharmacist was caught in the middle, prompting a leading health economist to predict that the "bloodiest new battle" in the ongoing managed-care war would "cut through the neighborhood pharmacy."[17]

Many pharmacists felt helpless when confronting angry patients complaining about their prescription prices. Some shrugged off the complaints by explaining that they were only passing on the costs they had to pay for the drugs; others suggested less expensive generic equivalents or therapeutic substitutes. For many patients, however, particularly senior citizens, the high cost of prescription medication was still intolerable. Those close to Canada organized bus trips across the border to purchase their prescriptions at governmentally controlled prices, placing even more pressure upon the American drug industry to justify their price structure. Does this economic issue present an ethical dilemma? What role does the individual pharmacist have in adjusting or controlling prescription drug prices?

### Case 5.12: Professional Responsibility in Controlling Prescription Prices

*"I didn't know I could do that."*

Pharmacist Jim Good has been practicing for nearly twenty years. He has increasingly been concerned about escalating drug prices, particularly for his elderly patients who constitute the bulk of his prescription business. Otto Bismarck, a retired auto worker, came in one morning with a prescription for an expensive drug designed to reduce his cholesterol level. Jim routinely consulted with his patients when physicians wrote for unusually expensive drugs. "The price of this prescription will be $100, but your drug plan will pick up only $25 of the cost," Jim said gently. "I'm afraid the doctor will want to keep you on this drug for some time." Mr. Bismarck looked crestfallen. "I can't afford this drug, Mr. Good. I'm on a limited income." Jim knows that Mr. Bismarck could probably not lower his cholesterol level by diet alone and asks, "Doesn't your union have a mail-order prescription plan?" Mr. Bismarck nodded. "I think so, but I've never tried it. It all seems so complicated. I didn't know I could do that." Jim knows that the union program will cover all but a fraction of Mr. Bismarck's prescription. Does Jim have an obligation to help Mr. Bismarck use the mail-order program to decrease his drug costs, even though he may not benefit personally from the transaction?

**Commentary:** The Code of Ethics for Pharmacists assures society that the pharmacist stands ready to "assist individuals in making the best use of medications" and to serve "individual, community, and society needs." Overarching this service component is the Code's expectation that the pharmacist "seeks justice in the distribution of health resources," attends to the "good of every patient in a caring, compassionate, and confidential manner," and relies on ethical principles "based on moral obligations and virtues." Collectively, these broad statements of purpose promise the patient that pharmaceutical services are far beyond mere transactional activities and that the pharmacist will see "the face of the one who suffers" and appreciate their singularity and uniqueness.[18] Assuring that the patient has access to needed medication is a primary duty of this level of pharmaceutical service.

Pharmacist Jim Good has encountered a common dilemma; Mr. Bismarck is confronted with a medication cost that poses a barrier to his treatment plan. Every stakeholder in the American health-care system, including the federal government and the pharmaceutical manufacturing industry, recognizes the difficult straits caused by the increasing cost of prescriptions. Even the promise of special discount plans for senior citizens and low-income families appears to offer little relief toward solving this problem. Still, pharmacist Good is facing Mr. Bismarck, and the situation begs an immediate response. To respond in a caring and compassionate manner will require dedication to an altruistic spirit and a sense of beneficence. Resolution of these kinds of challenges are generally dependent on the careful balancing of economic demands with strongly-held personal values, thus providing an opportunity for the virtuous pharmacist to meet the obligations of the Code of Ethics for Pharmacists.

### Case 5.13: Serving the Patient within the Boundaries of the Health-Care System

*"Doctor, I think we can save the hospital some money here"*

Pharmacist Joe Morrison was reviewing patient charts one morning and came across an alarming anomaly. Dr. Fischelis routinely prescribed an expensive anticoagulant to all his heart patients. Joe knew that coumadin therapy was much less expensive and provided equivalent benefit to all but a few refractory patients for whom there was a slight risk of hemorrhage. Joe's drug budget at the hospital had skyrocketed over the past few years and Joe felt obliged to cut costs where he could. Joe decided to discuss the issue with Dr. Fischelis personally. Joe laid out his therapeutic alternatives as clearly as he could. "Doctor, I think we can save the hospital some money here," he concluded. "Joe," Dr. Fischelis replied, "if there's the slightest risk to even one of my patients it's not worth it." Should Joe continue to pursue the issue? Do pharmacists bear some responsibility for controlling drug costs in an institutional setting or should they confine their advocacy to patient-related issues?

Commentary: The health-care system in the United States is currently dominated by corporate medical practices in both community and institutional settings. Large chain store operations are mushrooming on choice corner lots of American cities and towns, efficiently eliminating the small, privately operated pharmacy. Local hospitals, once a source of community pride, are combining with others to form megasystems that operate on an area- or state-wide basis; some hospital systems are even national in scope. As these medical care systems continue to increase in size and complexity, their operations increasingly perplex the patients they serve, and raise questions about excessive charges for prescription drugs.

The role of pharmacists in controlling the prices that patients have to pay for their medications is problematic, and yet pharmacists are constantly confronted with patients who are noticeably concerned about such costs. Too frequently, patients make public their claims about outrageous charges for their prescriptions, particularly from institutions where charges for medications may be many multiples of what they might encounter in a community pharmacy. Too often, the answer to such claims in the institutional environment is the standard justification, "but Medicare will only pay a part of it."

Ethically, pharmacist Joe Morrison must seek to do what is right as he confront these situations. Is health care a business or a responsibility, or is there a "moral hazard" present because some of his patients may have to pay large sums out-of-pocket since they are least likely to have trade-name versions prescribed than patients getting most of their costs reimbursed by a third party? Furthermore, Joe will need to remain alert and determine whether "the drug of choice" is the best-marketed drug or the drug with the best efficacy, side-effect profile, and cost-effectiveness. In all cases, Joe's actions should reflect the Code of Ethics for Pharmacists, allowing him to "seek justice in the distribution of health resources," promote fairness and equity, and attempt to balance "the needs of patients and society."

## Wrestling with the challenges of alternative medicines

Americans have always been fascinated with their personal health care. From the earliest days of the republic, the American public has ingested, applied, or inserted drug products into every available bodily orifice in search of relief from pain or maladies—either real or imagined. "Dosing" became a way of life for many Americans who saw self-care as an affirmation of a true democracy and were suspicious of medical practitioners who set themselves apart as a distinct profession. By the end of the nineteenth century, allopathic medicine had become the standard of care; other medical theories were either ridiculed or suppressed. A century later, alternative medicine has seen an amazing resurgence, fueled by high drug costs, impatience with physicians who could not provide a "quick fix" to chronic and often intractable diseases, and the challenge of multiculturalism.

Today, alternative medicine includes not only folk medicine practices from a variety of cultures, but other therapies outside the scope of generally accepted medical care, including acupuncture, aromatherapy, homeopathy, massage, reflexology, and bioelectro-magnetic devices. These therapies are often employed in conjunction with standard medical care; indeed, some 40 per cent of Americans use some form of complementary or alternative medicine, prompting the United States Congress to establish a center to examine and analyze alternative treatment therapies.

To pharmacists rigidly trained in the pharmaceutical sciences, many of these alternative therapies seemed incomprehensible or flew in the face of accepted medical science. Others saw the insatiable new demand for alternative medicines as an irresistible marketing opportunity and rode the crest of the wave of herbal medications that came to dominate the home care sections of many pharmacies. The drugs seemed harmless enough, they rationalized. Why not get in on the action? "After all, if I don't sell folks these drugs someone else will." Yet as studies revealing serious interactions between prescription medications and alternative therapies began to emerge, conscientious pharmacists could no longer afford to ignore therapies that could interfere with their patients' treatment plans, even if it meant confronting them with strongly held personal beliefs. What ethical responsibilities do pharmacists have when they are confronted with patients who may not benefit from alternative therapies? Do they intervene only when their patients face serious harm or do they actively attempt to change their patients' belief systems? The following cases provide some guidance to these thorny issues.

### Case 5.14: Dealing with Requests for Homeopathic Remedies

*"What do you think of this product?"*

Pharmacist Hank Whitney has a real quandary. His manager has insisted that he include a small section of homeopathic remedies in the self-care section of his pharmacy. Hank has absolutely no confidence in such remedies, which he considers the worst example of alternative medicines. Hank's personal beliefs do not allow him to recommend homeopathic remedies, but he forcefully states his beliefs whenever he receives request from patients, usually delicately inquiring how the patient acquired their beliefs. Mrs. Hahnemann bustles up to the prescription counter carrying a small vial of homeopathic granules of black cohosh. "What do you think of this product?" Mrs. Hahnemann inquires pleasantly. Hank replies that the drug had been used in Europe to treat symptoms of menopause, but there were many other drugs available which had proven efficacy. "Well, I was just wondering," Mrs. Hahnemann replied. "I've been taking it now for two years and it really seems to help my symptoms." Hank is aware that no long-term toxicity studies have been conducted on black cohosh. Does he have an ethical obligation to inform Mrs. Hahnemann about his concerns. Should Hank take a more active role in discouraging the use of homeopathic medicines?

**Commentary:**    Complementary and alternative medicine (CAM) is an area of great public interest and activity, both nationally and worldwide. Many alternative medical practices have existed for hundreds, even thousands of years. Patients and professionals who have found conventional medicine inadequate for a particular, usually chronic, medical condition are turning to CAM for a variety of reasons. Some are concerned about the side effects of conventional therapies; others are seeking out a more "holistic" orientation to their health care where they can address body, mind, and spirit.[19] These individuals are pursuing health outcomes that fit into a much wider range of health-care values.

Attempting to understand the ethical foundation for CAM practices will require pharmacists to go beyond the usual base of ethical theories such as principilism. One ethicist suggests that characteristics of both CAM and traditional medicine are embodied within such core values as integrated humanity, ecological integrity, naturalism, relationalism, and spiritualism.[20] These broad value statements need to be more deeply appreciated in order to apply them to this case. Ultimately, however, the situation will distill to a matter of Mrs. Hahnemann's autonomy, perhaps bounded by a duty not to harm. Pharmacist Hank Whitney will have to consider his role in "protecting the common good," especially in fulfilling his role as patient advocate by engaging in fruitful, open communication, including truthful personal thoughts about the requested drug product. He will need to assure himself that he is facilitating Mrs. Hahnemann's informed choice, and at the same time not advocating a harmful or useless practice.

### Case 5.15: Balancing Alternative and Rational Medicinal Practices

*"I've just about had it with this drug"*

Pharmacist Chuck Dohme is a conscientious practitioner in a small town in the Midwest. Recently, the Sunday paper published a feature article extolling the virtues of St. John's Wort for the treatment of depression. Chuck was prepared for some good-natured ribbing from his patients Monday morning, but he was not prepared when Sam Thomson stormed into his pharmacy and tossed an empty prescription vial of Prozac on the counter. "I've just about had it with this drug," Mr. Thomson complained. "It doesn't seem to do me any good. I might as well use this St. John's stuff I read about in the paper yesterday." Chuck is aware that St. John's Wort is widely used in Europe to treat depression, but comparative scientific studies with Prozac have so far been inconclusive. Should Chuck try to dissuade Mr. Thomson from using the herbal remedy? Should he urge him to continue his Prozac therapy? Should he refer Mr. Thomson to his physician? Is anyone harmed if Chuck takes no action at all?

**Commentary:**  The Code of Ethics for Pharmacists commits pharmacists to promoting the "good of every patient," a clear call for doing good and avoiding harm. Presumably, this concern for the health and well-being of the patient focuses on the mission of pharmaceutical care—to assist individuals in making the best use of their medications. With increased consumer awareness and personal preferences promoting the wide spread use of herbal remedies, pharmacists are more and more being confronted with decision-making opportunities that embody "doing good and avoiding harm." Using herbal products for various health reasons stands out as one of the most striking examples of world-wide alternative medical practice. Adventurous patients often engage in herbal therapy without the guidance of their physicians, combining herbs with their traditional medications, and even replacing them altogether. This case, a seemingly simple encounter between pharmacist and patient, demonstrates how complicated it can be for pharmacists to attempt to promote the well-being of their patients and promote the best use of their medications.

Pharmacist Chuck Dohme is faced with the challenge of balancing some questions that medical science has about the efficacy of St. John's Wort with his personal judgments concerning herbal therapy. On one hand, his considerable training in evidence-based medicine calls for the rigorous application of facts, yet his substantial experience with self-medication and the unexplainable outcomes of placebo therapy allows him leeway in deciding a course of action. Furthermore, because he realizes that evaluative judgments about alternative medical practices such as the use of herbal prod-

ucts are, at best, personal, he needs to confirm what health outcome Mr. Thomson is anticipating with his intended use of St.
John's Wort and decide if there is enough credible information
available to him to either reassure or discourage Mr. Thomson on
the use of the product. Chuck needs to answer Mr. Thomson's inquiry about St. John's Wort not only with a confident voice but
also with his strong recommendation for Mr. Thomson to include
his physician in the final decision.

## Concluding Remarks

As we have seen, the traditional responsibility of the practicing
pharmacist—the safe and efficient distribution of prescriptions and
other drug products—carries with it serious ethical responsibilities.
The time-honored physician-patient-pharmacist relationship that
characterized drug distribution during the first half of the twentieth century was both simple and direct, affording each participant
a certain sense of control. Decisions affecting the selection and
monitoring of drug therapy rarely extended beyond this triad.

The drug distribution system has expanded to involve a large
number of individuals and institutions, reflecting the realities of
pharmacy practice as it enters the new century—managed care systems, insurance programs, governmental mandates, nontraditional
marketing strategies, consumer demands, and other policies affect
the public's access and use of drugs and professional services. Decisions affecting drug therapy are no longer made independently, giving practitioners and patients alike a sense of loss of control: the
simple triad has become a polygon.

Moreover, because this system has evolved during a period of
sustained moral reflection, health-care practitioners now appear to
be committed to creating a health-care system solidly founded on
the tenets of social justice. This sense of social responsibility is also
exhibited in the virtue-based language of newly revised codes of
professional ethics. Pharmacists who embrace a professional practice that builds upon moral principles and virtues will find expanded opportunities for ethical decision-making as they strive to
meet the challenges of pharmaceutical care.

## Study Questions

5.1 Discuss the factors that contributed to the development of the modern drug distribution system. Which of these factors have ethical implications associated with them?

5.2 Which aspect of the current drug distribution system places the greatest constraints upon the autonomy of the pharmacist?

5.3 What moral principles and virtues underlie the issue of freedom of choice of drugs and services?

5.4 Describe the ethical foundation for: a) deciding ownership of prescription orders; b) granting senior citizen discounts; c) promoting drugs for off-label use; d) accepting direct-line faxed prescriptions; e) sponsoring direct-to-consumer advertising.

5.5 What ethical issues are associated with accepting additional discounts for agreeing to dispense only one manufacturer's generic line of drugs?

5.6 What important ethical concerns are associated with medicines produced with advanced biotechnology?

## Situations for Analysis

5.1 A major drug company has recently introduced a sustained-release dosage capsule of one of its drugs that is scheduled to go "off patent." The new capsule has no apparent therapeutic advantage over the older tablet version. In its attempt to maintain a competitive advantage, the drug company has instructed its medical service representatives to offer pharmacists a $5 bonus for every patient they are able to "switch" to the new capsule.

5.2 A large third-party processing corporation has offered you at no cost a new computerized dispensing system to replace your present system, which is badly outdated. In return, you must agree to allow the new system to automatically dump its dispensing data into the corporation's master compiler for subsequent analysis of physician prescribing patterns. The system has a safeguard that assures patient anonymity.

5.3 You are a pharmacist in a large hospital, specializing in IV admixture therapy. As a member of the pharmacy and therapeutics committee of your institution, you are asked to develop a policy which will reduce the hospital's exposure to lost revenues. You are asked to consider a proposal that restricts expensive TPN treatments only to patients who are covered by private insurance; under this policy, Medicare and Medicaid patients would receive a less costly therapy.

5.4 A child who was taken algae, melatonin, and valerian at home was admitted to your hospital. The family brought a supply of these items with them requested that the child be allowed to continue to use these products during his hospitalization. The physician, a pediatric resident, agreed to their request. Since these products were not on the hospital formulary, the nurse sent them to the pharmacy with the physician's medication order, requesting that they be processed for in-patient use. The hospital's policy on nonformulary products and medications brought into the hospital by patients requires the pharmacist to identify the products, approve their nonformulary use, and relabel them to hospital standards.

5.5 A pharmacist receives a prescription for 50 half-grain pentobarbital capsules to be labeled "take as directed" from a man whose wife suffers from incurable bone cancer and has fallen and broken her hip, causing constant, intractable pain. The man asks if his wife should take all the capsules at once. The pharmacist realizes that the woman intends to commit suicide with the assistance of her physician, a procedure which is legal in his state. What should the pharmacist say? Is there any ethical justification for refusing to fill such a prescription order?

# References

1. "Taking to the Streets," *Modern Healthcare 23*:17 (April 26, 1993), p. 48. While security guards kept the peaceful demonstration outside, PMA President Gerald Mossinghoff agreed to meet to discuss their demands, which included a price rollback and a five-year freeze on drug prices. *Ibid.*
2. "APhA Answers Questions About the Coordinated Care Network," *Pharmacy Today 32*:21 (October 11, 1993), p. 1. PAID Prescriptions, Inc., is owned by Medco Containment Services, Inc., one of the nation's largest mail-order prescription services. The controversy heated up considerably when Merck, a top-ranked pharmaceutical manufacturer, announced their intent to purchase Medco. The Community Retail Pharmacy Health Care Reform Coalition, representing NARD and the National Association of Chain Drug Stores, took offense that APhA

would presume to speak for retail pharmacists and endorse one particular mail-order prescription service. In 1994, recoiling from protests from state pharmaceutical associations and individual pharmacists alike, APhA quietly rescinded the agreement. See "The Coordinated Care Network: Myth Versus Fact," *Pharmacy Today 32*:22 (October 25, 1993), p. 1; and "Motion, September 15-18, 1994," pp. 75-76, APhA Foundation Archives, Washington, D.C.

3.   Elyse Tanouye, "Drug Makers Sued by Stores Over Pricing: Seven Firms Are Accused of Limiting Discounts," *The Wall Street Journal* (Eastern Edition) *222*:75 (October 15, 1992), p. A2. The action was brought by ten chains and ten independent pharmacies representing approximately ten per cent of community pharmacies nationwide.

4.   Jayne O'Donnell, "FTC Looks at Deals by Drugmakers," *USA Today* (September 30, 1999), p. 3B. Government officials were concerned that some brand-name pharmaceutical manufacturers were paying off generic manufacturers after suing them for patent infringement. Antitrust lawyer George Cary compared the deals to "getting run over by a car, suing the guy that hit you and then paying him and saying you settled the lawsuit." *Ibid.*

5.   Glenn Sonnedecker, *Kremers and Urdang's History of Pharmacy*, 4th ed., rev. (Philadelphia: J. B. Lippincott Company, 1976) p. 213. "Legally enforced standards and controls in any profession often have an ambivalent quality in the public mind," Sonnedecker states, noting the delicate balance between "the assurance of more predictable and effective professional services" and "the risk of fostering special privileges and restrictive practices that may not be in the public interest." *Ibid.*

6.   See Seth Landefeld, "The Rise of the Modern Hospital Idea: 1900-1913," *Synthesis: The Undergraduate Journal in the History and Philosophy of Science 1*:3 (October, 1973), p. 19. Hospital pharmacists became active in the APhA's Section on Practical Pharmacy and Dispensing, organizing their own Subsection on Hospital Pharmacy in 1936 and an independent American Society of Hospital Pharmacists in 1942.

7.   Paul C. Olson, "Marketing Drug Products," *Drug Trade News 34*:8 (April 6, 1959), p. 20. In 1931, American pharmacists dispensed 165 million prescriptions; by 1960, that figure had increased to 729 million prescriptions, representing a dollar volume of over $2.2 billion. Sonnedecker, *History of Pharmacy* (n. 5), pp. 312-13.

8.   See Don E. Francke, Clifton J. Latiolais, Gloria N. Francke, and Norman F. H. Ho, *Mirror to Hospital Pharmacy: A Report of the Audit of Pharmaceutical Services in Hospitals* (Washington, D.C.: American Society of Hospital Pharmacists, 1964), p. 36.

9.   See Lowell J. Anderson, "To Switch or Not to Switch?" *American Pharmacy NS34*:3 (March, 1994), p. 5; and "Minnesota Proposes Ethical Principles," *ibid.*, p. 15.

10.  Richard R. Abood and David B. Brushwood, *Pharmacy Practice and the Law* (Gaithersburg, Maryland: Aspen Publishers, Inc., 2001), p. 240.

11.  Sonnedecker, *History of Pharmacy* (n. 5), p. 314. Between 1964 and 1969, three different organizations developed or helped administer prepaid prescription insurance programs: PAID Prescriptions, Prepaid Prescription Plans, and Pharmaceutical Card System, Inc.

12.  *Ibid.*, p. 322. In the words of pharmacy historian Alex Berman, "the hospital formulary had now become the focal point for the control and

standardization of therapeutic agents; it reflected the policies of pharmacy and therapeutic committees; it prevented product duplication; it was a teaching aid; it helped set realistic drug inventories; and it was the product of progressive pharmacological knowledge." Alex Berman, "Historical Currents in American Hospital Pharmacy," *Drug Intelligence and Clinical Pharmacy 6*:12 (December, 1972), p. 443.

13. See, for example, "Metropolitan: Focusing on Health-Care Integration," *Drug Topics 137*:22 (November 22, 1993), pp. 38 and 43. At the time, Metropolitan's Medimet program had 50,000 pharmacies in its network (90 per cent of all pharmacies in the United States), utilizing a formulary managed by an outside consulting firm monitored by Medimet's own pharmacy and therapeutics committee.

14. "What is most profitable for the pharmacist will probably determine what drug the patient eventually gets," Columbia University's Harry Schwartz rails. Detecting "a whiff of possible corruption," Schwartz fantasizes about pharmacists directing patients to certain physicians in return for a portion of their fees. "Druggists and doctors may agree that the latter will write their prescriptions in a manner that will help the pharmacists earn the most dollars from PAID." Harry Schwartz, "The Shape of Things to Come," *Pharmaceutical Executive 13*:12 (December, 1993), p. 26. Also see n. 2 above.

15. Kathleen Marie Dixon and Karen L. Kier, "Longing for Mercy, Requesting Death: Pharmaceutical Care and Pharmaceutically Assisted Death," *American Journal of Health-System Pharmacy 55*:6 (March 15, 1998), pp. 578- 85.

16. Tatsuya Morita, Satoro Tsuneto, and Yasuo Shima, "Correspondence: Proposed Definitions for Terminal Sedation," *The Lancet 358*:9278 (July 28, 2001) pp. 335-36; and Daniel P. Sulmasy, Wayne A. Ury, Judith C. Ahronheim, Mark Siegler, Leon Kass, John Lantros, Robert A. Burt, Kathleen Foley, Richard Payne, Carlos Gomez, Thomas J. Krizek, Edmund D. Pellegrino, and Russell K. Portenoy, "Letters: Publication of Papers on Assisted Suicide and Terminal Sedation," *Annals of Internal Medicine 133*:7 (October 3, 2000), pp. 564-66.

17. J. D. Kleinke, "Just What the HMO Ordered: The Paradox of Increasing Drug Costs," *Health Affairs 19*:2 (March- April, 2000), p. 79.

18. Dixon and Kier, "Longing for Mercy, Requesting Death" (n. 15), p. 580.

19. Wayne B. Jonas, "Advising Patients on the Use of Complementary and Alternative Medicine," *Applied Psychophysiology and Biofeedback 26*:3 (September 26, 2001), pp. 205-14.

20. David E. Guin, "Ethics and Integrative Medicine: Moving Beyond the Biomedical Model," *Alternative Therapies in Health and Medicine 7*:6 (November-December, 2001), pp. 68-72.

## Suggested Readings

Brody, Howard. *The Healer's Power*. New Haven, Connecticut: Yale University Press, 1992.

Szasz, Thomas. *Our Right to Drugs: The Case for a Free Market*. Westport, Connecticut: Praeger, 1992.

Young, James Harvey. *The Medical Messiahs: A Social History of Health Quackery in Twentieth-Century America*. Princeton, New Jersey: Princeton University Press, 1967.

# Appendix A

# Codes of Ethics

 **Hippocratic Oath, 4th century, B.C.**[1]

I swear by Apollo Physician and Asclepius and Hygeia and Panacea and all the gods and goddesses, making them my witnesses, that I will fulfil according to my ability and judgment this oath and this covenant:

To hold him who has taught me this art as equal to my parents and to live my life in partnership with him, and if he is in need of money to give him a share of mine, and to regard his offspring as equal to my brothers in male lineage and to teach them this art—if they desire to learn it— without fee and covenant; to give a share of precepts and oral instruction and all other learning to my sons and to the sons of him who has instructed me and to pupils who have signed the covenant and have taken an oath according to the medical law, but to no one else.

I will apply dietetic measures for the benefit of the sick according to my ability and judgment; I will keep them from harm and injustice. I will neither give a deadly drug to anybody if asked for it, nor will I make a suggestion to this effect. Similarly, I will not give to a woman an abortive remedy. In purity and holiness I will guard my life and my art.

I will not use the knife, not even on sufferers from stone, but will withdraw in favor of such men as are engaged in this work.

Whatever houses I may visit, I will come for the benefit of the sick, remaining free from all intentional injustice, of all mischief and in particular of sexual relations with both female and male persons, be they free or slaves.

What I may see or hear in the course of the treatment or even outside of the treatment in regard to the life of men, which on no account one must spread abroad, I will keep to myself holding such things shameful to be spoken about.

If I fulfill this oath and do not violate it, may it be granted to me to enjoy life and art, be honored with fame among all men for all time to come; if I transgress it and swear falsely, may the opposite of all this be my lot.

# Philadelphia College of Pharmacy, 1848[2]

## Code of Ethics

Pharmacy being a profession which demands knowledge, skill, and integrity on the part of those engaged in it, and being associated with the medical profession in the responsible duties of preserving the public health, and dispensing the useful though often dangerous agents adapted to the cure of disease, its members should be united on some general principles to be observed in their several relations to each other, to the medical profession, and to the public.

The *Philadelphia College of Pharmacy* being a permanent, incorporated institution, embracing amongst its members a large number of respectable and well educated apothecaries, has erected a standard of scientific attainments, which there is a growing disposition on the part of candidates for the profession to reach; and being desirous, that in relation to professional conduct and probity, there should be a corresponding disposition to advance, its members having agreed upon the following principles for the government of their conduct:

1st. *The College of Physicians of Philadelphia* having declared that any connection with, or monied interest in apothecaries' stores, on the part of the physicians, should be discountenanced; *we in like manner consider* that an apothecary being engaged in furthering the interests of any particular physician, to the prejudice of other reputable members of the medical profession, or allowing any physician a percentage or commission on his prescriptions, as unjust toward that profession and injurious to the public.

2d. As the diagnosis and treatment of disease belong to the province of a distinct profession, and as a pharmaceutical education does not qualify the graduate for these responsible offices; we should, where it is practicable, refer applicants for medical aid to a regular physician.

3d. As the practice of Pharmacy can only become uniform, by an open and candid intercourse being kept up between apothecaries, which will lead them to discountenance the use of secret formulae, and promote the general use and knowledge of good practice, and as this College considers that any discovery which is useful in alleviating human suffering, or in restoring the diseased to health, should be made public for the good of humanity and the general advancement of the healing art,—no member of this College should originate or prepare a medicine, the composition of which is concealed from other members, or from regular physicians.

Whilst the College does not at present feel authorized to require its members to abandon the sale of secret or quack medicines, they earnestly recommend the propriety of discouraging their employment, when called upon for an opinion as to their merits.

4th. The apothecary should be remunerated by the public for his knowledge and skill, and his charges should be regulated by the time consumed in preparation, as well as by the value of the article sold; although location and other circumstances necessarily affect the rate of charges at different establishments, no apothecary should intentionally undersell his neighbors with a view to his injury.

5th. As medical men occasionally commit errors in the phraseology of their prescriptions, which may or may not involve ill consequences to the patient if dispensed, and be injurious to the character of the practitioner; it is held to be the duty of the apothecary, in such cases, to have the corrections made, if possible, without the knowledge of the patient, so that the physician may be screened from censure. When the errors are of such a character as not to be apparent, without the knowledge of circumstances beyond the reach of the apothecary, we hold him to be blameless in case of ill consequences, the prescription being his guarantee, the original of which should always be retained by the apothecary.

6th. Apothecaries are likewise liable to commit errors in compounding prescriptions,—*first*, from the imperfect handwriting of the physicians; *secondly*, owing to the various synonyms of drugs in use, and their imperfect abbreviations; *thirdly*, from the confusion which even in the best regulated establishments may sometimes occur, arising from press of business; and *fourthly*, from deficient knowledge or ability of one or more of the assistants in the shop, or of the proprietor—

We hold that in the first three instances named, it is the duty of the physician to stand between the apothecary and the patient, as far as possible; and in the last that he should be governed by the circumstances of the case—drawing a distinction between an error made by a younger assistant accidently engaged, and a case of culpable ignorance or carelessness in the superior.

7th. As the apothecary should be able to distinguish between good and bad drugs, in most cases, and as the substitution of a weak or inert drug for an active one, may, negatively, be productive of serious consequences—we hold that the intentional sale of impure drugs or medicines, from motives of competition, or desire of gain, when pure articles of the same kind may be obtained, is *highly culpable*, and it is the duty of every honest apothecary or druggist of expose all such fraudulent acts as may come to his knowledge. But in reference to those drugs which cannot be obtained in a state of purity, he should, as occasion offers, keep physicians informed of their quality, that they may be governed accordingly.

8th. As there are many powerful substances that rank as poisons, which are constantly kept by apothecaries, and prescribed by physicians, and which are only safe in their hands, as arsenious acid, vegetable alkaloids, ergot, cantharides, etc.—we hold that the apothecary is not justified in vending these powerful agents indiscriminately to persons unqualified to administer them, and that a prescription should always be required, except in those cases when the poisons are intended for the destruction of animals or vermin—and in these instances only with the guarantee of a responsible person. And we hold that when there is good reason to believe that the purchaser is habitually using opiates or stimulants to excess, every conscientious apothecary should discourage such practice.

9th. No apprentice to the business of apothecary should be taken for a less term than four years, unless he has already served a portion of that time in an establishment of good character. Apprentices should invariably be entered as matriculants in the school of pharmacy, and commence attendance on its lectures at least two years before the expiration of their term of apprenticeship; and as the progress of our profession in the scale of scientific attainment must depend mainly upon those who are yet to enter it—it is recommended that those applicants who have had the advantage of a good preliminary education, including the Latin language, should be preferred.

DANIEL B. SMITH, *President.*
CHARLES ELLIS, *1st Vice President.*
SAMUEL F. TROTH, *2d Vice President.*

*Attest,* DILLWYN PARRISH, *Secretary.*

# American Pharmaceutical Association, 1852[3]

## Code of Ethics

The American Pharmaceutical Association, composed of Pharmaceutists and Druggists throughout the United States, feeling a strong interest in the success and advancement of their profession in its practical and scientific relations, and also impressed with the belief that no amount of knowledge and skill will protect themselves and the public from the ill effects of an undue competition, and the temptations to gain at the expense of quality, unless they are upheld by high moral obligations in the path of duty, have subscribed to the following *Code of Ethics* for the government of their professional conduct.

ART. I. As the practice of pharmacy can only become uniform by an open and candid intercourse being kept up between apothecaries and druggists among themselves and each other, by the adoption of the National Pharmacopoeia as a guide in the preparation of official medicines, by the discontinuance of secret formulae and the practices arising from a quackish spirit, and by an encouragement of that *esprit de corps* which will prevent a resort to those disreputable practices arising out of an injurious and wicked competition;—*Therefore*, the members of this Association agree to uphold the use of the Pharmacopoeia in their practice; to cultivate brotherly feeling among the members, and to discountenance quackery and dishonorable competition in their business.

ART. II. As labor should have its just reward, and as the skill, knowledge and responsibility required in the practice of pharmacy are great, the remuneration of the pharmaceutist's services should be proportioned to these, rather than to the market value of the preparations vended. The rate of charges will necessarily vary with geographical position, municipal location, and other circumstances of a permanent character, but a resort to intentional and unnecessary reduction in the rate of charges among apothecaries, with a view to gaining at the expense of their brethren is strongly discountenanced by this Association as productive of evil results.

ART. III. The first duty of the apothecary, after duly preparing himself for his profession, being to procure good drugs and preparations, (for without these his skill and knowledge are of small avail,) he frequently has to rely on the good faith of the druggist for their selection: Those druggists whose knowledge, skill and integrity enable them to conduct their business faithfully, should be encouraged, rather than those who base their claims of patronage on the cheapness of their articles solely. When accidentally or otherwise, a deteriorated, or adulterated drug or medicine is sent to the apothecary, he should invariably return it to the druggist, with a statement of its defects. What is too frequently considered as a mere error of trade on the part of the druggist, becomes a *highly culpable* act when countenanced by the apothecary; hence, when repetitions of such frauds occur, they should be exposed for the benefit of the profession. A careful but firm pursuit of this course would render well-disposed druggists more careful and deter the fraudulently-inclined from a resort to their disreputable practices.

ART. IV. As the practice of pharmacy is quite distinct from the practice of medicine, and has been found to flourish in proportion as its practitioners have confined their attention to its requirements; and as the conduction of the business of both professions by the same individual involves pecuniary temptations which are often not compatible with a conscientious discharge of duty; we consider that the members of this Association should discountenance all such professional amalgamation; and in conducting business at the counter, should avoid prescribing for diseases when practicable, referring applicants for medical advice to the physician. We hold it as unprofessional and highly reprehensible for apothecaries to allow any per centage or commission to physicians on their prescriptions, as unjust to the public, and hurtful to the independence and self-respect of both the parties concerned. We also consider that the practice of some physicians, (in places where good apothecaries are numerous,) of obtaining medicines at low prices from the latter, and selling them to their patients, is not only unjust and unprofessional, but deserving the censure of all high minded medical men.

ART. V. The important influence exerted on the practice of pharmacy by the large proportion of physicians who have resigned its duties and emoluments to the apothecary, are reasons why he should seek their favorable opinion and cultivate their friendship, by earnest endeavors to furnish their patients with pure and well-prepared medicines. As physicians are liable to commit errors in writing their prescriptions, involving serious consequences to health and reputation if permitted to leave the shop, the apothecary should always, when he deems an error has been made, consult the physician before proceeding; yet in the delay which must necessarily occur, it is his duty, when possible, to accomplish the interview without compromising the reputation of the physician. On the other hand, when apothecaries commit errors involving ill consequences, the physician, knowing the constant liability to error, should feel bound to screen them from undue censure, unless the result of a culpable negligence.

ART. VI. As we owe a debt of gratitude to our predecessors for the researches and observations which have so far advanced our scientific art, we hold that every apothecary and druggist is bound to contribute his mite toward the same fund, by noting the new ideas and phenomena which may occur in the course of his business, and publishing them, when of sufficient consequence, for the benefit of the profession.

**American Pharmaceutical Association, 1922[4]**

## Code of Ethics

CHAPTER I.

*The Duties of the Pharmacist in Connection with His Services to the Public.*

Pharmacy has for its primary object the service which it can render to the public in safeguarding the handling, sale, compounding and dispensing of medicinal substances.

The practice of pharmacy demands knowledge, skill and integrity on the part of those engaged in it. Pharmacists are required to pass certain educational tests in order to qualify under the laws of our states. The states thus restrict the practice of pharmacy to those persons who by reason of special training and qualifications are able to qualify under regulatory requirements and grant to them privileges necessarily denied to others.

In return the states expect the Pharmacist to recognize his responsibility to the community and to fulfil his professional obligations honorably and with due regard for the physical and moral well-being of society.

The Pharmacist should uphold the approved legal standards of the United States Pharmacopoeia and the National Formulary for articles which are official in either of these works, and should, as far as possible, encourage the use of these official drugs and preparations and discourage the use of objectionable nostrums.[*] He should sell and dispense only drugs of the best quality for medicinal use and for filling prescriptions.

He should neither buy, sell nor use substandard drugs for uses which are in any way connected with medicinal purposes.

The Pharmacist should be properly remunerated by the public for his knowledge and skill when used in its behalf in compounding prescriptions, and his fee for such professional work should take into account the time consumed and the great responsibility involved as well as the cost of the ingredients.

The Pharmacist should not sell or dispense powerful drugs and poisons to persons not properly qualified to administer or use them, and

---

[*]An objectionable nostrum is one which does not meet the requirements of the definition of the Commission on Proprietary Medicines of the American Pharmaceutical Association.

should use every proper precaution to safeguard the public from poisons and from all habit-forming medicines.

The Pharmacist, being legally intrusted with the dispensing and sale of narcotic drugs and alcoholic liquors, should merit this responsibility by upholding and conforming to the laws and regulations governing the distribution of these substances.

The Pharmacist should seek to enlist and merit the confidence of his patrons and when this confidence is won it should be jealously guarded and never abused by extortion or misrepresentation or in any other manner.

The Pharmacist should consider the knowledge which he gains of the ailments of his patrons and their confidences regarding these matters, as entrusted to his honor, and he should never divulge such facts unless compelled to do so by law.

The Pharmacist should hold the health and safety of his patrons to be of first consideration; he should make no attempt to prescribe or treat diseases or strive to sell drugs or remedies of any kind simply for the sake of profit.

He should keep his pharmacy clean, neat and sanitary in all its departments and should be well supplied with accurate measuring and weighing devices and other suitable apparatus for the proper performance of his professional duties.

It is considered inimical to public welfare for the pharmacist to have any clandestine arrangement with any Physician in which fees are divided or in which secret prescriptions are concerned.

The Pharmacist should primarily be a good citizen, and should uphold and defend the laws of the state and nation. He should inform himself concerning the laws, particularly those relating to food and drug adulteration and those pertaining to health and sanitation and should always be ready to coöperate with the proper authorities having charge of the enforcement of the laws.

The Pharmacist should be willing to join any constructive effort to promote the public welfare and he should regulate his public and private conduct and deeds so as to entitle him to the respect and confidence of the community in which he practices.

CHAPTER II.

*The Duties of the Pharmacist in His Relations to the Physician.*

The Pharmacist even when urgently requested so to do should always refuse to prescribe or attempt diagnoses. He should, under such circumstances, refer applicants for medical aid to a reputable legally qualified Physician. In cases of extreme emergency as in accident or sudden illness on the street in which persons are brought to him pending the arrival of a Physician such prompt action should be taken to prevent suffering as is dictated by humanitarian impulses and guided by scientific knowledge and common sense.

The Pharmacist should not, under any circumstances, substitute one article for another, or one make of an article for another in a prescription, without the consent of the Physician who wrote it. No change should be made in a Physician's prescription except such as is essentially warranted by correct pharmaceutical procedure, nor any that will interfere with the obvious intent of the prescriber, as regards therapeutic action.

He should follow the Physician's directions explicitly in the matter of refilling prescriptions, copying the formula upon the label or giving a copy of the prescription to the patient. He should not add any extra directions or caution or poison labels without due regard for the wishes of the prescriber, providing the safety of the patient is not jeopardized.

Whenever there is doubt as to the interpretation of the Physician's prescription or directions, he should invariable confer with the Physician in order to avoid a possible mistake or an unpleasant situation.

He should never discuss the therapeutic effect of a Physician's prescription with a patron nor disclose details of composition which the Physician has withheld, suggesting to the patient that such details can be properly discussed with the prescriber only.

Where an obvious error or omission in a prescription is detected by the Pharmacist, he should protect the interests of his patron and also the reputation of the Physician by conferring confidentially upon the subject, using the utmost caution and delicacy in handling such an important matter.

CHAPTER III

*The Duties of Pharmacists to Each Other and to the Profession at Large.*

The Pharmacist should strive to perfect and enlarge his professional knowledge. He should contribute his share toward the scientific progress of his profession and encourage and participate in research, investigation and study.

He should associate himself with pharmaceutical organizations whose aims are compatible with this code of ethics and to whose membership he may be eligible. He should contribute his share of time, energy and expense to carry on the work of these organizations and promote their welfare. He should keep himself informed upon professional matters by reading current pharmaceutical and medical literature.

He should perform no act, nor should he be a party to any transaction, which will bring discredit to himself or to his profession or in any way bring criticism upon it, nor should he unwarrantedly criticize a fellow Pharmacist or do anything to diminish the trust reposed in the practitioners of pharmacy.

The Pharmacist should expose any corrupt or dishonest conduct of any member of his profession which comes to his certain knowledge, through those accredited processes provided by the civil laws or the rules and regulations of pharmaceutical organizations, and he should aid at driving the unworthy out of the calling.

He should not accept agencies for objectional nostrums nor allow his name to be used in connection with advertisements or correspondence for furthering their sale.

He should courteously aid a fellow Pharmacist who may request advice or professional information or who, in an emergency, needs supplies.

He should not aid any person to evade legal requirements regarding character, time or practical experience by carelessly or improperly endorsing or approving statements relating thereto.

He should not imitate the labels of his competitors nor take any other unfair advantage of merited professional or commercial success. When a bottle or package of a medicine is brought to him to be refilled, he should remove all other labels and place his own thereon unless the patron requests otherwise.

He should not fill orders which come to him by mistake, being originally intended for a competitor.

He should deal fairly with manufacturers and wholesale druggists from whom he purchases his supplies; all goods received in error or excess and all undercharges should be as promptly reported as are shortages and overcharges.

He should earnestly strive to follow all proper trade regulations and rules, promptly meet all obligations and closely adhere to all contracts and agreements.

# American Pharmaceutical Association, 1952[5]

## Code of Ethics

The primary obligation of pharmacy is the service it can render to the public in safeguarding the preparation, compounding, and dispensing of drugs and the storage and handling of drugs and medical supplies.

The practice of pharmacy requires knowledge, skill, and integrity; therefore, the state laws restrict the practice of pharmacy to persons with special training and qualifications and licenses to them privileges which are denied to others. Accordingly, the pharmacist recognizes his responsibility to the state and to the community for their well-being and fulfills his professional obligations honorably.

### *The Pharmacist and His Relations to the Public*

The pharmacist upholds the approved legal standards of the United States Pharmacopeia and the National Formulary, and encourages the use of official drugs and preparations. He purchases, compounds, and dispenses only drugs of good quality.

The pharmacist uses every precaution to safeguard the public when dispensing any drugs or preparations. Being legally intrusted with the dispensing and sale of these products, he assumes this responsibility by upholding and conforming to the laws and regulations governing the distribution of these substances.

The pharmacist seeks to enlist and merit the confidence of his patrons. He zealously guards this confidence. He considers the knowledge and confidence which he gains of the ailments of his patrons as entrusted honor, and he does not divulge such facts.

The pharmacist holds the health and safety of his patrons to be of first consideration; he makes no attempt to prescribe for or to treat disease or to offer for sale any drugs or medical device merely for profit.

The pharmacist keeps his pharmacy clean, neat, and sanitary, and well equipped with accurate measuring and weighing devices and other apparatus suitable for the proper performance of his professional duties.

The pharmacist is a good citizen and upholds and defends the laws of the states and nation; he keeps informed concerning pharmacy and drug laws, and other laws pertaining to health and sanitation, and cooperates with the enforcement authorities.

The pharmacist supports constructive efforts in behalf of the public health and welfare. He seeks representation on public health committees and projects and offers to them his full cooperation.

The pharmacist at all times seeks only fair and honest remuneration for his services.

## The Pharmacist in His Relations to the Other Health Professions

The pharmacist willingly makes available his expert knowledge of drugs to the other health professions.

The pharmacist refuses to prescribe or to diagnose; he refers those needing such service to a properly licensed practitioner. In an emergency and pending the arrival of a qualified practitioner, he applies such first-aid treatment as is dictated by humanitarian impulses, scientific knowledge, and good judgment.

The pharmacist compounds and dispenses prescriptions carefully and accurately, using correct pharmaceutical skill and procedure. If there is any question in the pharmacist's mind regarding the ingredients of a prescription, a possible error, or the safety of the direction, he privately and tactfully consults the practitioner before making any changes. He exercises his best professional judgment and follows, under the laws and existing regulations, the prescriber's directions in the matter of refilling prescriptions, copying the formula upon the label, or giving a copy of the prescription to the patient. He adds any extra directions or caution or poison labels only with proper regard for the wishes of the prescriber, and the safety of the patient.

The pharmacist does not discuss the therapeutic effect or composition of a prescription with a patient. When such questions are asked, he suggests that the qualified practitioner is the proper person with whom such matters should be discussed.

The pharmacist considers it inimical to public welfare to have any clandestine arrangement with any practitioner of the health sciences by which fees are divided or in which secret or coded prescriptions are involved.

## The Pharmacist and His Relations to Fellow Pharmacists

The pharmacist strives to perfect and enlarge his professional knowledge. He contributes his share toward the scientific progress of his profession and encourages and participates in research, investigation, and study. He keeps himself informed regarding professional matters by reading current pharmaceutical, scientific, and medical literature, attending seminars and other means.

The pharmacist seeks to attract to his profession youth of good character and intellectual capacity and aids in their instruction.

The pharmacist associates himself with organizations having for their objective the betterment of the pharmaceutical profession and contributes his share of time, energy, and funds to carry on the work of these organizations.

The pharmacist keeps his reputation in public esteem by continuously giving the kind of professional service that earns its own reward. He does not engage in any activity or transaction which will bring discredit or criticism to himself or to his profession.

The pharmacist will expose any corrupt or dishonest conduct of any member of his profession which comes to his certain knowledge, through those accredited processes provided by the civil laws or the rules and regulations of pharmaceutical organizations, and he will aid in driving the unworthy out of the calling.

The pharmacist does not lend his support or his name to the promotion of objectionable or unworthy products.

The pharmacist courteously aids a fellow pharmacist who may request advice or professional information or who, in an emergency, may need supplies.

The pharmacist does not imitate the labels of his competitors or attempt to take any unfair advantage of their professional or commercial success. He does not fill orders that he knows are intended for a competitor. He deals fairly with manufacturers and wholesalers and recognizes the significance and legal aspects of brand names and trade-marked products. He adheres to fair business practices, meets his obligations promptly, and fulfills his agreements and contracts.

The pharmacist is proud to display in his establishment his own name and the names of other pharmacists employed by him.

**American Pharmaceutical Association, 1969[6]**

### Code of Ethics

**Preamble.** These principles of professional conduct for pharmacists are established to guide the pharmacist in his relationship with patients, fellow practitioners, other health professionals and the public.

**Section 1.** A pharmacist should hold the health and safety of patients to be of first consideration; he should render to each patient the full measure of his ability as an essential health practitioner.

**Section 2.** A pharmacist should never knowingly condone the dispensing, promoting or distributing of drugs or medical devices, or assist therein, which are not of good quality, which do not meet standards required by law or which lack therapeutic value for the patient.

**Section 3.** A pharmacist should always strive to perfect and enlarge his professional knowledge. He should utilize and make available this knowledge as may be required in accordance with his best professional judgment.

**Section 4.** A pharmacist has the duty to observe the law, to uphold the dignity and honor of the profession, and to accept its ethical principles. He should not engage in any activity that will bring discredit to the profession and should expose, without fear or favor, illegal or unethical conduct in the profession.

**Section 5.** A pharmacist should seek at all times only fair and reasonable remuneration for his services. He should never agree to, or participate in transactions with practitioners of other health professions or any other person under which fees are divided or which may cause financial or other exploitation in connection with the rendering of his professional services.

**Section 6.** A pharmacist should respect the confidential and personal nature of his professional records; except where the best interest of the patient requires or the law demands, he should not disclose such information to anyone without proper patient authorization.

**Section 7.** A pharmacist should not agree to practice under terms or conditions which tend to interfere with or impair the proper exercise of his professional judgment and skill, which tend to cause a deterioration of the quality of his service or which require him to consent to unethical conduct.

Section 8. A pharmacist should not solicit professional practice by means of advertising or by methods inconsistent with his opportunity to advance his professional reputation through service to patients and to society.

Section 9. A pharmacist should associate with organizations having for their objective the betterment of the profession of pharmacy; he should contribute of his time and funds to carry on the work of these organizations.

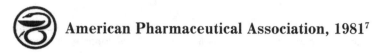

# American Pharmaceutical Association, 1981[7]

## Code of Ethics

### Preamble

These principles of professional conduct are established to guide pharmacists in relationships with patients, fellow practitioners, other health professionals, and the public.

A **Pharmacist** should hold the health and safety of patients to be of first consideration and should render to each patient the full measure of professional ability as an essential health practitioner.

A **Pharmacist** should never knowingly condone the dispensing, promoting, or distributing of drugs or medical devices, or assist therein, that are not of good quality, that do not meet standards required by law, or that lack therapeutic value for the patient.

A **Pharmacist** should always strive to perfect and enlarge professional knowledge. A pharmacist should utilize and make available this knowledge as may be required in accordance with the best professional judgment.

A **Pharmacist** has the duty to observe the law, to uphold the dignity and honor of the profession, and to accept its ethical principles. A pharmacist should not engage in any activity that will bring discredit to the profession and should expose, without fear or favor, illegal or unethical conduct in the profession.

A **Pharmacist** should seek at all times only fair and reasonable remuneration for professional services. A pharmacist should never agree to, or participate in, transactions with practitioners of other health professions or any other person under which fees are divided or that may cause financial or other exploitation in connection with the rendering of professional services.

A **Pharmacist** should respect the confidential and personal nature of professional records; except where the best interest of the patient requires or the law demands, a pharmacist should not disclose such information to anyone without proper patient authorization.

A **Pharmacist** should not agree to practice under terms or conditions that interfere with or impair the proper exercise of professional judgment and skill, that cause a deterioration of the quality of professional services, or that require consent to unethical conduct.

A **Pharmacist** should strive to provide information to patients regarding professional services truthfully, accurately, and fully and should avoid misleading patients regarding the nature, cost, or value of these professional services.

A **Pharmacist** should associate with organizations having for their objective the betterment of the profession of pharmacy and should contribute time and funds to carry on the work of these organizations.

**American Pharmaceutical Association, 1994**[8]

### Code of Ethics for Pharmacists

Pharmacists are health professionals who assist individuals in making the best use of medications. This Code, prepared and supported by pharmacists, is intended to state publicly the principles that form the fundamental basis of the roles and responsibilities of pharmacists. These principles, based on moral obligations and virtues, are established to guide pharmacists in relationships with patients, health professionals, and society.

I.　**A pharmacist** respects the covenantal relationship between the patient and pharmacist.

Considering the patient-pharmacist relationship as a covenant means that a pharmacist has moral obligations in response to the gift of trust received from society. In return for this gift, a pharmacist promises to help individuals achieve optimum benefit from their medications, to be committed to their welfare, and to maintain their trust.

II.　**A pharmacist** promotes the good of every patient in a caring, compassionate, and confidential manner.

A pharmacist places concern for the well-being of the patient at the center of professional practice. In doing so, a pharmacist considers needs stated by the patient as well as those defined by heath science. A pharmacist is dedicated to protecting the dignity of the patient. With a caring attitude and a compassionate spirit, a pharmacist focuses on serving the patient in a private and confidential manner.

III.　**A pharmacist** respects the autonomy and dignity of each patient.

A pharmacist promotes the right of self-determination and recognizes individual self-worth by encouraging patients to participate in decisions about their health. A pharmacist communicates with patients in terms that are understandable. In all cases, a pharmacist respects personal and cultural differences among patients.

IV.　**A pharmacist** acts with honesty and integrity in professional relationships.

A pharmacist has a duty to tell the truth and to act with conviction of conscience. A pharmacist avoids discriminatory practices, behavior or work conditions that impair professional judgment, and actions that compromise dedication to the best interests of patients.

V.       **A pharmacist** maintains professional competence.

A pharmacist has a duty to maintain knowledge and abilities as new medications, devices, and technologies become available and as health information advances.

VI.      **A pharmacist** respects the values and abilities of colleagues and other health professionals.

When appropriate, a pharmacist asks for the consultation of colleagues or other health professionals or refers the patient. A pharmacist acknowledges that colleagues and other health professionals may differ in the beliefs and values they apply to the care of the patient.

VII.     **A pharmacist** serves individual, community, and societal needs.

The primary obligation of a pharmacist is to individual patients. However, the obligations of a pharmacist may at times extend beyond the individual to the community and society. In these situations, a pharmacist recognizes the responsibilities that accompany these obligations and acts accordingly.

VIII.    **A pharmacist** seeks justice in the distribution of health resources.

When health resources are allocated, a pharmacist is fair and equitable, balancing the needs of patients and society.

*This code was approved by the membership of the American Pharmaceutical Association on October 27, 1994.*

## American Medical Association

Physicians dedicated to the health of America

## American Medical Association, 2001[9]

### Principles of Medical Ethics

### Preamble

The medical profession has long subscribed to a body of ethical statements developed primarily for the benefit of the patient. As a member of this profession, a physician must recognize responsibility to patients first and foremost, as well as to society, to other health professionals, and to self. The following Principles adopted by the American Medical Association are not laws, but standards of conduct which define the essentials of honorable behavior for the physician.

I.      A physician shall be dedicated to providing competent medical care with compassion and respect for human dignity and rights.

II.     A physician shall uphold the standards of professionalism, be honest in all professional interactions, and strive to report physicians deficient in character or competence, or engaging in fraud or deception, to appropriate entities.

III.    A physician shall respect the law and also recognize a responsibility to seek changes in those requirements which are contrary to the best interests of the patient.

IV.     A physician shall respect the rights of patients, colleagues, and other health professionals, and shall safeguard patient confidences and privacy within the constraints of the law.

V.      A physician shall continue to study, apply, and advance scientific knowledge, maintain a commitment to medical education, make relevant information available to patients, colleagues, and the public, obtain consultation, and use the talents of other health professionals when indicated.

VI.     A physician shall, in the provision of appropriate patient care, except in emergencies, be free to choose whom to serve, with whom to associate, and the environment in which to provide medical care.

VII. A physician shall recognize a responsibility to participate in activities contributing to the improvement of the community and the betterment of public health.

VIII. A physician shall, while caring for a patient, regard responsibility to the patient as paramount.

IX. A physician shall support access to medical care for all people.

## Fundamental Elements of the Patient-Physician Relationship

From ancient times, physicians have recognized that the health and well-being of patients depends upon a collaborative effort between physician and patient. Patients share with physicians the responsibility for their own health care. The patient-physician relationship is of greatest benefit to patients when they bring medical problems to the attention of their physicians in a timely fashion, provide information about their medical condition to the best of their ability, and work with their physicians in a mutually respectful alliance. Physicians can best contribute to this alliance by serving as their patients' advocate and by fostering these rights:

1. The patient has the right to receive information from physicians and to discuss the benefits, risks, and costs of appropriate treatment alternatives. Patients should receive guidance from their physicians as to the optimal course of action. Patients are also entitled to obtain copies or summaries of their medical records, to have their questions answered, to be advised of potential conflicts of interest that their physicians might have, and to receive independent professional opinions.

2. The patient has the right to make decisions regarding the health care that is recommended by his or her physician. Accordingly, patients may accept or refuse any recommended medical treatment.

3. The patient has the right to courtesy, respect, dignity, responsiveness, and timely attention to his or her needs.

4. The patient has the right to confidentiality. The physician should not reveal confidential communications or information without the consent of the patient, unless provided for by law or by the need to protect the welfare of the individual or the public interest.

5. The patient has the right to continuity of health care. The physician has an obligation to cooperate in the coordination of medically indicated care with other health care providers treating the patient. The

physician may not discontinue treatment of a patient as long as further treatment is medically indicated, without giving the patient sufficient opportunity to make alternative arrangements for care.

6. The patient has a basic right to have available adequate health care. Physicians, along with the rest of society, should continue to work toward this goal. Fulfillment of this right is dependent on society providing resources so that no patient is deprived of necessary care because of an inability to pay for the care. Physicians should continue their traditional assumption of a part of the responsibility for the medical care of those who cannot afford essential health care. Physicians should advocate for patient in dealing with third parties when appropriate.

American Nurses Association, 2001[10]

### Code of Ethics for Nurses

1.  The nurse, in all professional relationships, practices with compassion and respect for the inherent dignity, worth, and uniqueness of every individual, unrestricted by considerations of social or economic status, personal attributes, or the nature of health problems.

2.  The nurse's primary commitment is to the patient, whether an individual, family, group, or community.

3.  The nurse promotes, advocates for, and strives to protect the health, safety, and rights of the patient.

4.  The nurse is responsible and accountable for individual nursing practice and determines the appropriate delegations of tasks consistent with the nurse's obligation to provide optimum patient care.

5.  The nurse owes the same duties to self as to others, including the responsibility to preserve integrity and safety, to maintain competence, and to continue personal and professional growth.

6.  The nurse participates in establishing, maintaining, and improving health care environments and conditions of employment conducive to the provision of quality health care and consistent with the values of the profession through individual and collective action.

7.  The nurse participates in the advancement of the profession through contributions to practice, education, administration, and knowledge development.

8.  The nurse collaborates with other health professionals and the public in promoting community, national, and international efforts to meet health needs.

9.  The profession of nursing, as represented by associations and their members, is responsible for articulating nursing values, for maintaining the integrity of the profession and its practice, and for shaping social policy.

# AHA    American Hospital Association, 1992[11]

## A Patient's Bill of Rights

*Introduction*

Effective health care requires collaboration between patients and physicians and other health care professionals. Open and honest communication, respect for personal and professional values, and sensitivity to differences are integral to optimal patient care. As the setting for the provision of health services, hospitals must provide a foundation for understanding and respecting the rights and responsibilities of patients, their families, physicians, and other caregivers. Hospitals must ensure a health care ethic that respects the role of patients in decision making about treatment choices and other aspects of their care. Hospitals must be sensitive to cultural, racial, linguistic, religious, age, gender, and other differences as well as the needs of persons with disabilities.

The American Hospital Association presents a Patient's Bill of Rights with the expectation that it will contribute to more effective patient care and be supported by the hospital on behalf of the institution, its medical staff, employees, and patients. The American Hospital Association encourages health care institutions to tailor this bill of rights to their patient community by translating and/or simplifying the language of this bill of rights as may be necessary to ensure that patients and their families understand their rights and responsibilities.

*Bill of Rights*

These rights can be exercised on the patient's behalf by a designated surrogate or proxy decision maker if the patient lacks decision-making capacity, is legally incompetent, or is a minor.

1.   The patient has the right to considerate and respectful care.

2.   The patient has the right and is encouraged to obtain from physicians and other direct caregivers relevant, current, and understandable information concerning diagnosis, treatment, and prognosis.

     Except in emergencies when the patient lacks decision-making capacity and the need for treatment if urgent, the patient is entitled to the opportunity to discuss and request information related to the specific pro-

cedures and/or treatments, the risks involved, the possible length of re-
cuperation, and the medically reasonable alternatives and their accom-
panying risks and benefits.

Patients have the right to know the identity of physicians, nurses, and
others involved in their, as well as when those involved are students,
residents, or other trainees. The patient also has the right to know the
immediate and long-term financial implications of treatment choices
insofar as they are known.

3.   The patient has the right to make decisions about the plan of care prior
     to and during the course of treatment and to refuse a recommended
     treatment or plan of care to the extent permitted by law and hospital
     polity and to be informed of the medical consequences of this action. In
     case of such refusal, the patient is entitled to other appropriate care and
     services that the hospital provides or transfer to another hospital. The
     hospital should notify patients of any policy that might affect patient
     choice within the institution.

4.   The patient has the right to have a advance directive (such as a living
     will, health care proxy, or durable power of attorney for health care)
     concerning treatment or designating a surrogate decision maker with
     the expectation that the hospital will honor the intent of that directive
     to the extent permitted by law and hospital policy.

     Health care institutions must advise patients of their rights under state
     law and hospital policy to make informed medical choices, ask if the
     patient has an advance directive, and include that information about
     hospital policy that may limit its ability to implement fully a legally
     valid advance directive.

5.   The patient has the right to every consideration of privacy. Case discus-
     sion, consultation, examination, and treatment should be conducted so
     as to protect each patient's privacy.

6.   The patient has the right to expect that all communications and records
     pertaining to his/her care will be treated as confidential by the hospital,
     except in cases such as suspected abuse and public health hazards when
     reporting is permitted or required by law. The patient has the right to
     expect that the hospital will emphasize the confidentiality of this infor-
     mation when it releases it to any other parties entitled to review infor-
     mation in these records.

7.   The patient has the right to review the records pertaining to his/her
     medical care and to have the information explained or interpreted as
     necessary, except as restricted by law.

8. The patient has the right to expect that, within its capacity and policies, a hospital will make reasonable response to the request of a patient for appropriate and medically indicated care and services. The hospital must provide evaluation, service, and/or referral as indicated by the urgency of the case. When medically appropriate or legally permissible, or when a patient has so requested, a patient may be transferred to another facility. The institution to which the patient is to be transferred must first have accepted the patient for transfer. The patient must also have the benefit of complete information and explanation concerning the need for, risks, benefit, and alternatives to such a transfer.

9. The patient has the right to ask and be informed of the existence of business relationships among the hospital, educational institutions, other health care providers, or payers that may influence the patient's treatment and care.

10. The patient has the right to consent or decline to participate in proposed research studies or human experimentation affecting care or treatment or requiring direct patient involvement, and to have those studies fully explained prior to consent. A patient who declines to participate in research or experimentation is entitled to the most effective care that the hospital can otherwise provide.

11. The patient has the right to expect reasonable continuity of care when appropriate and to be informed by physicians and other caregivers of available and realistic patient care option when hospital care is no longer appropriate.

12. The patient has the right to be informed of hospital policies and practices that relate to patient care, treatment, and responsibilities. The patient has the right to be informed of available resources for resolving disputes, grievances, and conflicts, such as ethics committees, patient representatives, or other mechanisms available in the institution. The patient has the right to be informed of the hospital's charges for services and available payment methods.

The collaborative nature of health care requires that patients, or their families/surrogates, participate in their care. The effectiveness of care and patient satisfaction with the course of treatment depend, in part, on the patient fulfilling certain responsibilities. Patients are responsible for providing information about past illnesses, hospitalizations, medications, and other matters related to health status. To participate effectively in decision making, patients must be encouraged to take responsibility for requesting additional information or clarification about their health status or treatment when the do not fully understand information and instructions. Patients are also responsible for ensuring that the health care institution has a copy of their written advance directive if they have one. Patients are responsible for informing their physicians and other caregivers if they anticipate problems in following prescribed treatment.

Patients should also be aware of the hospital's obligation to be reasonably efficient and equitable in providing care to other patients and the community. The hospital's rules and regulations are designed to help the hospital meet this obligation. Patients and their families are responsible for making reasonable accommodations to the needs of the hospital, other patients, medical staff, and hospital employees. Patients are responsible for providing necessary information for insurance claims and for working with the hospital to make payment arrangements, when necessary

A person's health depends on much more than health care services. Patients are responsible for recognizing the impact of their life-style on their personal health.

*Conclusion*

Hospitals have many functions to perform, including the enhancement of health status, health promotion, and the prevention and treatment of injury and disease; the immediate and ongoing care and rehabilitation of patients; the education of health professionals, patients, and the community; and research. All these activities must be conducted with an overriding concern for the values and dignity of patients.

**National Association of Boards of Pharmacy, 1992**[12]

Pharmacy Patient's Bill of Rights

## PREAMBLE

IN ACKNOWLEDGMENT of an increasingly informed and cost-conscious public, and with specific reference to the proliferation and complexity of drug therapy, Pharmacists have recognized the need for a "Pharmacy Patient's Bill of Rights." To reinforce their commitment to protect the health and well-being of their patients, Pharmacists need a common reference to describe their covenantal relationship with the public. In recognition of the public's right to freedom of choice and the Pharmacists' professional relationship with their patients, this document delineates: 1) the patient's rights and responsibilities with respect to appropriate drug therapy, and 2) the patient's responsibilities and Pharmacist's rights with respect to the quality of services provided. Such as charter is set forthwith and shall be known as the "Pharmacy Patient's Bill of Rights."

## PATIENT RIGHTS/PHARMACIST'S RESPONSIBILITIES

**Patients have the right to expect their pharmacist to:**

1. Be professionally competent and adhere to accepted standards of pharmacy practice.

2. Treat them with dignity, consistent with professional standards for all patients, regardless of manner of payment, race, sex, age, nationality, religion, disability, or other discriminatory factors.

3. Act in their best interest when making pharmaceutical care decisions.

4. Serve as their advocate for appropriate drug therapy and to make reasonable efforts to recommend alternative choices in coordination with the patients' other health care providers.

5. Maintain their medical records, keeping them confidential, using them routinely to maximize their care and making them available to the patient for review upon request.

6. Provide counseling, using the methods appropriate to the patients' physical, psychosocial, and intellectual status.

7.  Have their prescriptions dispensed and pharmacy services provided at a pharmacy of their choice in an atmosphere which allows for confidential communication and in an environment which is private, properly lighted, well-ventilated, and clean.

8.  Monitor drug therapy within their medical regimen for safety and efficacy and make reasonable efforts to detect and prevent drug allergies, adverse drug reactions, contraindications, or inappropriate dosage.

9.  Monitor their compliance and proper drug use and institute remedial interventions when necessary.

10. Prominently post the Pharmacy Patient's Bill of Rights.

## PATIENT RESPONSIBILITIES/PHARMACIST'S RIGHTS

**In order for pharmacists to meet their responsibilities to patients as set forth in this "Pharmacy Patient's Bill of Rights," patients are responsible for:**

1.  Providing the personal demographics, medical history, and payment mechanism including third party payor information necessary for Pharmacists to individualize care, the method of its provision, and its reimbursement.

2.  Implementing the drug therapy regimen conscientiously and reporting their clinical response to their pharmacist, especially untoward reactions and any changes in their health status and medical care.

3.  Cooperating with the pharmacist and authorizing their physician or other health care practitioner to release the medical information necessary for the pharmacist to practice responsibly.

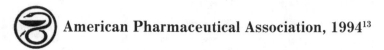 **American Pharmaceutical Association, 1994**[13]

### Pledge of Professionalism

As a student of pharmacy, I believe there is a need to build and reinforce a professional identity founded on integrity, ethical behavior and honor. This development, a vital process in my education, will help to ensure that I am true to the professional relationship I establish between myself and society as I become a member of the pharmacy community. Integrity will be an essential part of my everyday life and I will pursue all academic and professional endeavors with honesty and commitment to service.

To accomplish this goal of professional development, as a student of pharmacy I will:

A.    DEVELOP a sense of loyalty and duty to the profession by contributing to the well-being of others and by enthusiastically accepting the responsibility and accountability for membership in the profession.

B.    FOSTER professional competency through life-long learning. I will strive for high ideals, teamwork, and unity within the profession in order to provide optimal patient care.

C.    SUPPORT my colleagues by actively encouraging personal commitment to the Oath of a Pharmacist and the Code of Ethics for Pharmacists as set forth by the profession.

D.    DEDICATE my life and practice to excellence. This will require an ongoing assessment of personal and professional values.

E.    MAINTAIN the highest ideals and professional attributes to insure and facilitate the covenantal relationship required of the pharmaceutical care giver.

The profession of pharmacy is one that demands adherence to a set of ethical principles. These high ideals are necessary to insure the quality of care extended to the patients I serve. As a student of pharmacy, I believe this does not start with graduation; rather, it begins with my membership in this professional college community. Therefore, I will strive to uphold this pledge as I advance toward full membership in the profession.

I voluntarily make this pledge of professionalism.

# References

1. Ludwig Edelstein, "The Hippocratic Oath: Text, Translation and Interpretation," in *Ancient Medicine: Selected Papers of Ludwig Edelstein*, edited by Owsei Temkin and C. Lilian Temkin (Baltimore: Johns Hopkins University, 1967), p. 6. The so-called "Pagan Oath of Hippocrates" was translated by W. H. S. Jones from an attempted reproduction of the *textus receptus* of medieval times, based on Marcianus Venetus 269, fol. 12 (11th c. MSS in Venice), Vaticanus Greacus 276, fol. 1 (12th c. MSS in the Vatican), and Vaticanus Graecus 299, fol. 25 (14th c. MSS in the Vatican). Jones also translated the "Cruciform Oath" given in Urbinus 64, fol. 116 (10th or 11th c. MS in the Vatican), the oldest extant form of the Oath, modified "Insofar as a Christian May Swear It." See Chauncey D. Leake, *Percival's Medical Ethics* (Baltimore: The Williams & Wilkins Company, 1927), pp. 213-17.

2. "A Code of Ethics Adopted by the Philadelphia College of Pharmacy," *American Journal of Pharmacy 20*:2 (April, 1848), pp. 148-51. "If the Quaker apothecaries had done nothing else of moment this code would remain as a monument to the lofty principles which actuated these men who were not simply theorists, but who carried into their daily work the idealism which they held up as a pattern to their professional brethren." Charles H. LaWall, "Pharmaceutical Ethics: A Historical Review of the Subject with Examples of Codes Adopted or Suggested at Different Periods, Together with a Suggested Code for Adoption by Present-Day Associations," *Journal of the American Pharmaceutical Association 10*:11 (November, 1921), p. 898.

3. "Code of Ethics of the American Pharmaceutical Association," *Proceedings of the National Pharmaceutical Convention, Held at Philadelphia, October 6th, 1852* (Philadelphia: Merrihew & Thompson, Printers, 1852), pp. 24-26.

4. "Code of Ethics of the American Pharmaceutical Association (Adopted August 17, 1922)," *Journal of the American Pharmaceutical Association 11*:9 (September, 1922), pp. 728-29. The original draft appears in Charles H. LaWall, "Pharmaceutical Ethics," *ibid. 10*:12 (December, 1921), pp. 961-63.

5. "Code of Ethics of the American Pharmaceutical Association," *Journal of the American Pharmaceutical Association* (Practical Pharmacy Edition) *13*:10 (October, 1952), pp. 721-23. The Code was characterized as "a statement of principles adopted by the profession for the self-government of its members." *Ibid.*, p. 721.

6. "APhA Code of Ethics," *Journal of the American Pharmaceutical Association NS9*:11 (November, 1969), p. 552.

7. "Code of Ethics, American Pharmaceutical Association" [approved by active and life members, August, 1969; amended December, 1975; revised July, 1981], from a placard issued by the Association. Also see "APhA Code of Ethics," *Journal of the American Pharmaceutical Asso-*

*ciation NS9*:11 (November, 1969), p. 552. Section 8 of the 1969 Code, "A pharmacist should not solicit professional practice by means of advertising or by methods inconsistent with his opportunity to advance his professional reputation through service to patients and society," was amended in 1975 to be more circumspect of the federal antitrust laws and revised again in 1981 to remove all references to gender. See "Membership Votes Approval of Changes in Constitution, Bylaws, Code of Ethics," *APhA Weekly 15*:3 (January 17, 1976), p. 1, and "Code of Ethics, American Pharmaceutical Association," *ibid. 15*:40 (October, 1976), p. 3.

8.  Code of Ethics Review Committee, "Proposed: Code of Ethics for Pharmacists," *American Pharmacy NS34*:8 (August, 1994), p. 79. A placard issued later by the Association does not include the Committee's commentary on each principle.

9.  Adopted by the American Medical Association's House of Delegates, June 17, 2001. See American Medical Association Council on Ethical and Judicial Affairs, *Code of Medical Ethics Supplement* (July, 2001), p. i. Also see "Opinion: Update for Patient Advocacy: Principles of Medical Ethics," *American Medical News 44*:30 (August 13, 2001), p. 26; American Medical Association Council on Ethical and Judicial Affairs, *Code of Medical Ethics: Current Opinions with Annotation, 1994 Edition* (Chicago: American Medical Association, 1994), pp. xxxiv-xxxv. For a short historical development of the AMA Code of Ethics, see *ibid.*, pp. ix-x. Earlier versions of the Code may be found in Chauncey D. Leake, *Percival's Medical Ethics* (Baltimore: The Williams & Wilkins Company, 1927), pp. 218-38 [1847], 239-56 [1903], and 257-71 [1912].

10.  American Nurses Association, *Code of Ethics for Nurses with Interpretive Statements* (Washington, D.C.: American Nurses Association, 2001), p. 4. A "Code for Professional Nurses," containing 17 provisions, was adopted by the Association in 1950 and has been revised periodically. *Ibid.*, p. 27. Also see ANA Code of Ethics Project Task Force, "Issues Update: A New Code of Ethics for Nurses: Combining an Unchanged Mission with the Challenges of Contemporary Nursing," *American Journal of Nursing 100*:7 (July, 2000), pp. 69, 71-72; and "HOD Takes Bold Steps to Shape Direction of Nursing, ANA," *The American Nurse 33*:4 (July-August, 2001), p. 8.

11.  American Hospital Association, *A Patient's Bill of Rights* (Chicago: American Hospital Association, 2001). The Bill of Rights was first adopted by the American Hospital Association in 1973; this revision was approved by its Board of Trustees on October 21, 1992.

12.  "Pharmacy Patient's Bill of Rights," *U.S. Pharmacist 17*:5 (May, 1992), p. 68. Also see Hind T. Hatoum, "Pharmacy's Stake in the Patient's Bill of Rights," *ibid.*, pp. 60-62, 64 ,66-67, 88; Carmen A. Catizone, "NABP's Role in Developing a Bill of Rights," *ibid.*, p. 70; and "NABP Develops Pharmacy Patient's Bill of Rights," *NABP Newsletter 21*:5 (June, 1992), pp. 49, 51.

13.  The "Pledge of Professionalism" was adapted from a pledge developed

by the University of Illinois College of Pharmacy in 1993 and adopted
by the American Pharmaceutical Association Academy of Students and
the American Association of Colleges of Pharmacy Council of Deans
Task Force on Professionalism on June 26, 1994. From a placard issued
by the Association.

# APPENDIX B

# *FACIES PRO CAUSIS*[*]

Case 2.1:    *Daniel B. Smith* of Philadelphia was a founder of the Philadelphia College of Pharmacy (1821) and the first President of the American Pharmaceutical Association (1852-53).

*Dr. Thomas Bond* of Philadelphia, in association with Benjamin Franklin, secured funds in 1752 to establish the Pennsylvania Hospital, the first hospital in the United States.

Case 2.2:    *Rev. Henry Soloman Lehr* of Ada, Ohio, was the founder of Ohio Northern University (1871).

*William A. Brewer* of Boston was the second President of the American Pharmaceutical Association (1853-54).

Case 2.3:    *William B. Chapman* of Cincinnati was the third President of the American Pharmaceutical Association (1854-55).

*Dr. Elisha Perkins* of Connecticut secured the first United States patent for an electro-galvanic medical device in 1796. His so-called "metallic tractors" were supposed to draw noxious electrical fluid from the body when stroked across the skin.

Case 2.4:    *Margaret Sanger* of Corning, New York, was an influential leader in the birth-control movement in the United States in the early twentieth century.

*John Meakim* of New York was the fourth President of the American Pharmaceutical Association (1855-56).

*George W. Andrews* of Baltimore was the fifth President of the American Pharmaceutical Association (1856-57).

Case 2.5:    *Charles Ellis* of Philadelphia was the sixth President of the American Pharmaceutical Association (1857-58).

*Rev. Thomas R. Malthus*, English economist and sociologist, a pioneer of modern population study, warned in 1803 that the world's food supply would be outstripped by population growth unless tempered by sexual restraint, stimulating the first interest in controlling overpopulation through birth control.

---

[*] Roughly translated, "The Faces for the Cases."

Case 2.6:   *John L. Kidwell* of Georgetown, D.C., was the seventh President of the American Pharmaceutical Association (1858-59).
*Samuel M. Colcord* of Boston was the eighth President of the American Pharmaceutical Association (1859-60).
*Dorothea L. Dix* of Hampden, Maine, one of the greatest social reformers of the nineteenth century, succeeded in getting the insane out of jails and orphans out of almshouses.

Case 3.1:   *Henry T. Kiersted* of New York was the ninth President of the American Pharmaceutical Association (1860-61).

Case 3.2:   *Elizabeth Marshall* of Philadelphia is generally considered America's first woman pharmacist. In 1804, she took over the management of the professional apothecary shop established by her grandfather, Christopher Marshall in 1729.
*Zada M. Cooper* of Iowa was founder of Kappa Epsilon Pharmacy Fraternity for women, Secretary of the American Association of Colleges of Pharmacy (1922-42), and the first (and only) female President of Rho Chi Pharmacy Honor Society (1938-40).
*J. Faris Moore* of Baltimore was the eleventh President of the American Pharmaceutical Association (1863-64).

Case 3.3:   *William Procter, Jr.* of Philadelphia, one of the most eminent of American pharmacists, was the first professor of pharmacy at the Philadelphia College of Pharmacy (1846), editor of the *American Journal of Pharmacy* (1850-71), and the tenth President of the American Pharmaceutical Association (1863-64).

Case 3.4:   *Lydia E. Pinkham* of Massachusetts, a prominent nineteenth-century feminist and abolitionist, developed a famous Vegetable Compound for all types of female complaints composed of unicorn root, pleurisy root, and other herbs in an 18 per cent alcohol base.
*William J. M. Gordon* of Cincinnati was the twelfth President of the American Pharmaceutical Association (1864-65).

Case 3.5:   *Alexis St. Martin* of Mackinac Island, Michigan, suffered an accidental gunshot wound to his stomach in 1822 and was successfully treated by Dr. William Beaumont.
*Dr. William Beaumont*, an early nineteenth-century army surgeon, carried out a long series of carefully planned experiments on Alexis St. Martin through a permanent stomach fistula resulting from a gunshot wound. The publication of these classic

experiments in 1833 provided the first insight into the chemical nature of gastric digestion.

*Henry W. Lincoln* of Boston was the thirteenth President of the American Pharmaceutical Association (1865-66).

Case 3.6:     *Frederick Stearns* of Detroit was the fourteenth President of the American Pharmaceutical Association (1866-67).

*James M. Munyon* of Scranton, Pennsylvania, founder of the Munyon Homeopathic Home Remedy Company in the late nineteenth century, advertised that he had a "Munyon pill for every ill," and claimed to be able to cure asthma, catarrh, rheumatism, and a host of other complaints.

Case 3.7:     *Jonathan Swift*, eighteenth-century English satirist and clergyman, suffered a lingering and degrading death, experiencing pain so intense that knives had to be kept out of his reach.

*John Milhau* of New York was the fifteenth President of the American Pharmaceutical Association (1867-68).

Case 3.8:     *Edward Parrish* of Philadelphia, Professor of Pharmacy at the Philadelphia College of Pharmacy, also established a "School of Practical Pharmacy" in 1843 as an important adjunct to his professional practice and was the sixteenth President of the American Pharmaceutical Association (1868-69).

*Annie Besant* and Charles Bradlaugh were tried in England in 1877 for selling *The Fruits of Philosophy*, a pamphlet on contraceptive methods written in 1832 by Charles Knowlton. Their trial prompted the founding of the Malthusian League, an early advocate of birth control.

Case 3.9:     *Dr. Richard C. Cabot*, a turn-of-the-century physician and early critic of the usual practice of "benevolent deception" in medical practice, advocated telling the absolute truth to his patients, foreshadowing the concept of informed consent.

*Ezekiel H. Sargent* of Chicago was the seventeenth President of the American Pharmaceutical Association (1869-70).

Case 3.10:    *Richard H. Stabler* of Alexandria, Virginia, was the eighteenth President of the American Pharmaceutical Association (1870-71).

*John Farr* of Philadelphia, a founder of the Philadelphia College of Pharmacy, established John Farr & Company in 1818, an early manufacturer of medicinal and other chemicals, which was absorbed into Merck and Company of New York in 1927.

Case 4.1:     *Enno Sander* of St. Louis was the nineteenth President of the American Pharmaceutical Association (1871-72) and Honorary President of the Association from 1909 to 1910.

*Marie Sklodowska Curie*, a Polish physicist and chemist, worked with her husband, Pierre, to discover radium in 1898.

Case 4.2:     *Mary Putnam Jacoby* is generally considered to be the first woman to graduate with a degree in pharmacy. She graduated from the New York College of Pharmacy in 1863.

*"Lethe Rivers"* refers to the Lethe River in Greek mythology, the river of forgetfulness whose water produced loss of memory in those who drank it.

*Albert E. Ebert* of Chicago was Professor of Professor at the Chicago College of Pharmacy and the twentieth President of the American Pharmaceutical Association (1872-73). He is commemorated by the Ebert Prize for Pharmaceutical Research.

Case 4.3:     *John F. Hancock* of Baltimore was the twenty-first President of the American Pharmaceutical Association (1873-74).

*Dr. John Redman Coxe* of Philadelphia was Professor of Medicine at the University of Pennsylvania and author of the *American Dispensatory* (1806).

*Mrs. Winslow's Soothing Syrup* was a particularly notorious example of the patent medicines of the late nineteenth century. The syrup contained a large percentage of alcohol and morphine, and was suggested for use in babies suffering the pains of colic and teething.

Case 4.4:     *Cotton Mather*, American clergyman and author, and Fellow of the Royal Society, encouraged physicians to inoculate against smallpox during a Boston epidemic in 1721.

*C. Lewis Diehl* of Louisville, Kentucky, was the twenty-second President of the American Pharmaceutical Association (1874-75).

Case 4.5:     *George F. H. Markoe* of Boston was the twenty-third President of the American Pharmaceutical Association (1875- 76).

Case 4.6:     *Louise Baker* received her certificate from the Massachusetts College of Pharmacy in 1877, and was one of the first women to graduate from an association-based college of pharmacy.

*Stuart Craddock*, a laboratory assistant of Sir Alexander Fleming, became the first person to benefit from penicillin therapy by allowing Fleming to flush his infected sinuses with a dilute penicillin broth in 1929.

*Sir Alexander Fleming*, Scottish bacteriologist and physician, was the co-discoverer of penicillin (1929), for which he received the Nobel Prize in medicine in 1945.

Case 4.7:    *Charles Bullock* of Philadelphia was the twenty-fourth President of the American Pharmaceutical Association (1876- 77).
*Lutz Small* and his coworkers conducted basic chemical research on the morphine molecule in 1929 in an attempt to reduce its addictive properties.
*Thomas de Quincy* wrote *Confessions of an Opium Eater* in 1821, a semifictional account of the experiences of drug addicts.

Case 4.8:    *Mary Upjohn* was an 1871 graduate of the University of Michigan College of Pharmacy, one of the first women to graduate from a public college of pharmacy.
*Digitalis Lanata* is one of several varieties of *Scrophulariaceae* used to stimulate the beat of the heart.
*William Withering*, an eighteenth-century English physician, botanist, and social reformer who introduced digitalis into orthodox medicine following his studies of the use of foxglove in treating dropsy.

Case 4.9:    *William Saunders* of London, Ontario, was the twenty-fifth President of the American Pharmaceutical Association (1877-78).
*Gustavus J. Luhn* of Charleston, South Carolina, was the twenty-sixth President of the American Pharmaceutical Association (1878-79).

Case 4.10:   *James T. Shinn* of Philadelphia was an 1854 graduate of Philadelphia College of Pharmacy and the twenty-eighth President of the American Pharmaceutical Association (1880-81).
*George W. Sloan* of Indianapolis was the twenty-seventh President of the American Pharmaceutical Association (1879-80).
*Carry Nation* was an American temperance agitator of the early twentieth century who supplemented public prayers and denunciation by the personal destruction of property in saloons with a hatchet.

Case 4.11:   *P. Wendover Bedford* of New York was the twenty-ninth President of the American Pharmaceutical Association (1881-82).
*Charles A. Heinitsh* of Lancaster, Pennsylvania, was the thirtieth President of the American Pharmaceutical Association (1882-83).
*Dr. Theodore C. Janeway* published the first treatise on human blood pressure in the United States, *The Clinical Study of Blood Pressure: A Guide to the Use of the Sphygmomanometer* (1904), in which he introduced the term "essential hypertension."

Case 4.12:   *William S. Thompson* of Washington, D.C., was the thirty-first President of the American Pharmaceutical Association (1883-84).

*Claude Hopkins*, generally regarded as the "Father of Scientific Advertising," once wrote copy for Dr. Shoop's Patent Medicine Company of Racine, Wisconsin.

**Case 4.13:** *Edward C. Kendall* received the Nobel Prize in 1950 for his pioneering work on the hormones of the adrenal gland cortex and investigated the use of cortisone in the treatment of rheumatoid arthritis.

*John Ingalls* of Macon, Georgia, was the thirty-second President of the American Pharmaceutical Association (1884-85).

**Case 4.14:** *Joseph Roberts* of Baltimore was the thirty-third President of the American Pharmaceutical Association (1885-86).

*Karl Paul Link*, a biochemist at the University of Wisconsin, isolated dicumarol from sweet clover in 1940.

**Case 5.1:** *Virginia Dare* was the first child born of English parents in the Western Hemisphere, on Roanoke Island on the North Carolina coast in 1587.

*Alexander Graham Bell* discovered the principle of telephonic transmission while experimenting with a multiple harmonic telegraph in 1875. He introduced the telephone to the world in 1876 at the Philadelphia Centennial Exposition.

*Charles A. Tufts* of Dover, New Hampshire, was the thirty-fourth President of the American Pharmaceutical Association (1886-87).

**Case 5.2:** *C. Rufus Rorem* and Robert P. Fischelis authored *The Costs of Medicines* as part of the 1932 Report of the Costs of Medical Care, an early study of the economics of the American health-care system.

*John Uri Lloyd* of Cincinnati was a pharmaceutical manufacturer, chemist, teacher, author of both scientific literature and novels, and the thirty-fifth President of the American Pharmaceutical Association (1887-88).

**Case 5.3:** *Sir Rowland Hill* proposed reforms in the English postal service, including universal penny postage prepaid by adhesive postage stamps or official envelopes, a system adopted in 1839 and begun the following year.

*Maurice W. Alexander* of St. Louis was the thirty-sixth President of the American Pharmaceutical Association (1888-89).

**Case 5.4:** *Rexford G. Tugwell* was Under Secretary of Agriculture under President Franklin D. Roosevelt and a former Professor of Economics at Columbia University who led an unsuccessful battle to control drug advertising in the mid-1930s.

*Emlen Painter* of New York was the thirty-seventh President of the American Pharmaceutical Association (1889-90).

Case 5.5: *Alice Braunworth Halstead* established a record in 1928 for the longest continuous membership in the American Pharmaceutical Association of any woman to that time; she joined the Association in 1892.

*Dr. Arthur C. Christie* helped write a minority report which vigorously opposed the corporatization of medical practice, a position supported by the Committee on the Costs of Medical Care (1932) upon which he served.

*Dr. Ray Lyman Wilbur* was Chairman of the Committee on the Costs of Medical Care (1932), the first comprehensive socioeconomic study of the American health-care system.

Case 5.6: *Alfred B. Taylor* of Philadelphia was one of the earliest American pharmacists to combine practical pharmacy with scientific work; he served as the first Treasurer (1852-54) and thirty-eighth President of the American Pharmaceutical Association (1890-91).

*Philo T. Farnsworth* was an American inventor whose work on electronic imaging tubes in the 1920s led to the development of cathode-ray tubes used in television transmission.

Case 5.7: *Alexander K. Finlay* of New Orleans was the thirty-ninth President of the American Pharmaceutical Association (1891-92).

*Marie Carmichael Stopes*, early twentieth-century English eugenist, founded the first birth-control clinic in the British Empire, giving impetus to similar movements elsewhere.

Case 5.8: *Joseph P. Remington* was Dean of the Philadelphia College of Pharmacy, author of *Remington's Practice of Pharmacy*, and the fortieth President of the American Pharmaceutical Association (1892-93).

*Dr. William Gregory* of Edinburgh suggested a new process for obtaining morphine to Pierre Jean Robiquet in 1821, resulting in Robiquet's discovery of codeine.

*Pierre Jean Robiquet* ("Roby Kaye"), nineteenth-century French pharmacist and phytochemist, discovered many important natural chemicals, including codeine, caffeine, and amygdalin.

Case 5.9: *Susan Hayhurst* had charge of the pharmacy of the Woman's Hospital of Philadelphia for nearly three decades during the mid-nineteenth century.

*Dr. Edward C. Dodds* discovered the estrogenic hormone stilbestrol in 1938, the first synthetic substance to be employed for the control of cancer.

Case 5.10: *Edgar L. Patch* of Boston was the forty-first President of the American Pharmaceutical Association (1893-94).
*Emile Durkheim* authored an early sociological study of suicide, *Suicide* (1951).
*Dr. Karl A. Menninger* authored an early psychoanalytic study of suicide, *Man Against Himself* (1938).

Case 5.11: *William Simpson* of Raleigh, North Carolina was the forty-second President of the American Pharmaceutical Association (1894-95).
*Jean-Martin Charcot* (1825-93), Chair for the Study of Nervous Disorders at France's Saltêpetrière Clinic, was the first to describe amyotrophic lateral sclerosis, initially named Charcot's Disease in his honor.
*Henry Louis "Lou" Gehrig* (1903-41), first baseman for the New York Yankees, played 2,130 consecutive games before succumbing to amyotrophic lateral sclerosis, which was named "Lou Gehrig's Disease" in his memory.

Case 5.12: *James M. Good* of St. Louis was the forty-third President of the American Pharmaceutical Association (1895-96).
*Otto von Bismarck* (1815-98), first chancellor of the modern German empire, despite violent opposition, ensured the passage of sweeping legislation providing for sickness, accident, and old-age insurance.

Case 5.13: *Joseph E. Morrison* of Montreal, Canada was the forty-fourth President of the American Pharmaceutical Association (1896-97).
C. Rufus Rorem and *Robert P. Fischelis* authored *The Costs of Medicines* as part of the 1932 Report of the Costs of Medical Care, an early study of the economics of the American healthcare system.

Case 5.14: *Henry M. Whitney* of Lawrence, Massachusetts was the forty-fifth President of the American Pharmaceutical Association (1897-98).
*Samuel Christian Frederich Hahnemann* (1755-1843), German physician and chemist, founded the theory and practice of homeopathy.

Case 5.15: *Charles E. Dohme* of Baltimore was the forty-sixth President of the American Pharmaceutical Association (1898-99).
*Samuel Thomson* (1769-1843) founded the American botanic school of medical thought, which was later merged into the eclectic school of medicine.

# Appendix C

## GLOSSARY[*]

These notes are supplementary to the topics of the text and are intended to assist the interested reader in broadening their appreciation of the multiple issues presented throughout the chapters.

**Altruism.** The principle or practice of unselfish concern for or devotion to the welfare of others.

**Antisubstitution laws.** State-based legislation passed in the early 1950s making it illegal for a pharmacist to dispense a different brand of a prescription drug for the branded drug prescribed without obtaining the prescriber's prior approval. With the advent of bioequivalent generic drugs, the expansion of both government-based and private health insurance plans, the growth of HMOs, much of this legislation was repealed; by 1978, 40 states had repealed their antisubstitution legislation.

**APhA Judicial Board.** The body empowered by the American Pharmaceutical Association to receive and resolve complaints filed against individual members for unprofessional conduct. The Board may discipline members by reprimand, suspension, or expulsion. In addition, the Board may render advisory opinions and interpretive statements on matters of ethical pharmacy practice.

**Applied ethics.** The use of ethical theory and the methods of ethical analysis to examine ethical questions in the practice of the professions, technology use, and public policy.

**Assisted suicide.** Ending one's own life with the help of another person.

**Autonomy.** An action-guiding moral principle obliging us to respect the particular decisions of adults with decision-making capacity. Derived from

---

[*] Some terms in this Glossary are adapted from Raymond J. Devettere, *Practical Decision Making in Health Care Ethics: Cases and Concepts*, 2nd ed. (Washington, D.C.: Georgetown University Press, 2000), pp. 620-28, *passim*. Also see Richard Hedges, *Bioethics, Health Care, and the Law: A Dictionary* (Santa Barbara, California: ABC-CLIO, Inc., 1999); and Warren Thomas Reich, ed., *Encyclopedia of Bioethics*, rev. ed. (New York: Simon & Schuster Macmillan, 1995), 5 vols.

the Greek *autos* (self) and *nomos* (rule or law), this principle requires
recognition of the right of individuals to determine their own future
without interference from others. Also called the "right of self-determination" or the "right of self-rule."

**Beneficence.** An action-guiding moral principle obliging us to help others
and to promote their welfare. Derived from the Latin *bene* (well; from
*bonus*, good) and *facere* (to do), this principle follows the principle of
autonomy in priority and complements the principle of nonmaleficence
by prioritizing patients' right to services in their best interest and becomes dominant when patients are unable or incompetent to communicate their personal choices.

**Bestowed rights.** Rights that are granted by others, such as a government, an
institution, or an individual. Such rights may include the right to a living wage, the right to privacy, or the right to health care.

**CAM.** Complementary and alternative medicine. Those medical practices,
systems, interventions, and applications that currently are not part of
the dominant or conventional medical system. The group includes over
300 different topics.

**C. Douglas Hepler.** Professor of Pharmacy Health Care Administration at
the University of Florida College of Pharmacy. One of the early proponents of pharmaceutical care as a philosophy of professional pharmacy
practice.

**Capitation.** A payment system whereby providers agree in advance the cost
for providing care for a number of persons (the "head count") for a specified period, regardless of how much care they might have to provide in
response to their patients' needs.

**Caring.** Compassionate concern for an individual expressed by cognitively
learned humanistic behavior that protects and preserves the health, welfare, and human dignity of another individual. A moral duty or obligation for individuals in certain relationships to others, such as the relationship between pharmacists and patients.

**Casuistry.** A method of analyzing and resolving instances of moral perplex-
ity by interpreting general moral roles in light of particular circumstances. As particular moral questions (or "cases") are resolved, the resolutions gradually fit into typical patterns or categories, which then serve
as models for resolving similar cases, not unlike the appeal to prior cases
by lawyers and judges in legal proceedings. Derived from the Latin *ca-
sus* (event, occasion, occurrence, and later, case).

**Code of Ethics for Pharmacists.** The most widely accepted code of ethics for pharmacists in the United States. It was developed by the American Pharmaceutical Association and accepted by its members October 27, 1994.

**Code of ethics.** A formal statement by a group that establishes and prescribes moral and nonmoral standards and behaviors for members of that group.

**Consequentialism.** Any moral philosophy holding that actions are right or wrong according to the balance of their good or bad consequences. The right act in any circumstance is the one that produces the best overall result, as determined from an impersonal perspective that gives equal weight to the interests of each affected party. *Act consequentialism* requires agents to perform the particular action that in a particular situation is most likely to maximize good consequences; *rule consequentialism* requires agents to follow those moral rules the observance of which will maximize good consequences. Utilitarianism is the most prominent consequence-based ethical theory.

**Correlativity of rights.** The notion that for every claimed right there is a corresponding obligation or duty, or for an obligation there will be a corresponding right . For example, for the claim of a right to life, the moral system (or the legal system) imposes an obligation on others not to deprive the claimant of life. If a pharmacist accepts John Doe as a patient and delivers medication and advice, the pharmacist accepts an obligation and John Doe gains correlative rights. This notion of correlativity, however, is labeled by some scholars as "untidy," meaning that situations do exist where the right/obligation correlativity is unclear, perhaps nonexistent.

**Counter-prescribing.** A practice whereby a pharmacist goes beyond the role of dispenser of medication and provides treatment information and medication for an illness as perceived and presented by a patient. Such practices have been labeled as unethical by both the medical and pharmacy profession, however, nineteenth- and early twentieth-century medical practices encouraged apothecaries (pharmacists) to treat patients in this manner. Current pharmacy practice acts in some states allow pharmacists to "counter-prescribe."

**Covenant.** An agreement, usually formal, between two or more persons to do or not do something specified. In its ancient and most influential form, a covenant usually included the following elements: an original experience of gift between the soon-to-be covenanted partners; a covenant promise based on this original or anticipated exchange of gifts, labors, or services; and the shaping of subsequent life for each partner by the promissory event. This model carries an element of professional gratitude that pushes the health professional to go beyond the bare minimum of what may be agreed upon in a contract-based relationship.

**Deduction.** In moral philosophy, deduction is the reasoning process that applies a general moral principle or rule, or a right considered to be possessed by everyone, to a particular situation in order to determine what ought to be done. The deductivist model regards the action-guiding function of ethical theory to be the development of highly abstract and general first principles that, together with some factual description of a particular morally problematic situation, will entail concrete action guides. Moral principles developed and defended within normative ethical theory will play the role of premises in deductive arguments for ethical judgments about particular cases. See **Induction**.

**Deontology.** Any moral philosophy based on duty. Traditional deontological theories are moralities of law (divine law, natural law, or the moral law we give ourselves). Right-based theories can also be deontological in that one person's natural right creates a duty on the part of others to respect. Deontological theories usually propose a set of absolute duties or prohibitions; that is, certain actions are always and everywhere immoral regardless of good intentions, extenuating circumstances, or favorable circumstances. Modern deontology treats moral obligations as requirements that bind us to act, in large measure, independent of the effects our actions may have on our own good or well-being, and to a substantial extent, event independent of the effects of our actions on the well-being of others. For example, people have a moral imperative to tell the truth. Maintaining truthfulness makes society a better place where people are able to relate to one another with trust, resulting in a quality human experience; consequences are not an issue.

**DNA.** Desoxyribonucleic acid, the chemical thread in each cell carrying genetic instructions for that organism.

**Double effect.** A principle developed centuries ago by moral theologians to justify, under certain conditions, performing actions that have bad as well as good effects. In some cases, it produces moral judgments everyone is happy with, such as cases for those opposed to abortion when it is used to justify the medically necessary removal of a cancerous uterus despite the loss of an early fetus. In other cases, it produces moral judgments practically nobody is happy with, such as cases where some theologians might require the medically unnecessary removal of the site of an ectopic pregnancy whenever an ectopic pregnancy is terminated. Sometimes abbreviated as PDE (principle of double effect).

**DRG.** Diagnosis-related group. A classification system based primarily on diagnosis but adjusted for other factors. The DRG determines what the federal government will reimburse providers for services provided to Medicare-eligible patients.

**Durham-Humphrey Amendment (1951).** Federal legislation which established the classification of prescription-legend drugs which may be dispensed only by a written or oral prescription and whose refilling is authorized in the original prescription or by oral order of a practitioner. This Amendment had the effect of reversing the traditional professional prerogative of pharmacists to monitor their patients' medication use.

**Duty.** The responsibility or obligation of one person to another. The duty of care entails providing services to patients at the prevailing clinical standard, which must equal the national standard of quality of care. The bestowed right of health-care assistance to the indigent through Medicaid implies an obligation to all pharmacists to provide that assistance in an equitable manner. Physicians have a duty to warn others in cases where a patient informs the physician of his or her intent to harm others and a duty to warn their patients of problems associated with the medications they prescribe. See **Informed Consent.**

**Equity.** The quality or ideal of being just, fair, or impartial.

**Ethical pharmaceuticals.** The term "ethical specialty" was coined in 1876 by Detroit drug manufacturer Frederick Stearns to distinguish his line of simple preparations sold directly to the public, bearing full directions for use and the names and quantities of their ingredients. The term "ethical pharmaceutical" was later used to distinguish manufactured drug products promoted to the medical profession from those promoted directly to the public.

**Ethical assumptions.** The supposition that one or more moral principles are inherent to a particular ethical dilemma. For example, a pharmacist who chooses always to tell the truth operates on the ethical assumption that all pharmacists are honest and trustworthy and would never lie to their patients.

**Ethical outrage.** Situations in which the claim for right action is condemned by all. The pharmacist who defends fraudulent welfare billing on the basis of sluggish claims processing may be termed an ethical outrage.

**Ethics of care.** A distinctive form of moral reasoning which places great emphasis on beneficence as the health-care provider's primary responsibility to individual patients; a type of virtue ethic that focuses on the affective orientation and moral commitment of the one who cares. The ethics of care emphasize ethical actions rooted in a contextual understanding of specific situations, and focuses on such rudimentary moral skills as kindness, sensitivity, attentiveness, tact, patience, and reliability. The healing relationship is one of inherent inequality because patients are vulnerable and ill. In light of the patients' diminished power, health-care providers incur a duty of beneficence requiring them to satisfy their patients' needs, promote their good, and enhance their autonomy. An ethic of care suggests both a feeling response directed to individual patients and a commitment to ensure that things go well for them.

**Euthanasia.** A term coined by Sir Francis Bacon, drawn from the Greek *eu* (good or noble) and *thantos* (death), literally, "a good death." The term is ordinarily used to describe the intentional killing of a patient by a physician. *Active euthanasia* is the direct killing or ending of someone's life by any method such as lethal injection or a lethal dose of medication. *Passive euthanasia* is the withholding or withdrawing of a life-sustaining measure in order to allow a person to die.

**Fair dealing.** Being fair and equitable in professional and business dealings with patients and other members of the health-care team.

**Faithfulness.** A firm, undeviating loyalty to a person, cause, or idea. See Fidelity.

**FFS.** Fee-for-service payment system. Pharmacists or others provide services to patients then bill the patients or third-party payers for the services.

**Fidelity.** An ethical principle that obliges us to remain faithful to our commitments, especially in keeping promises and the protection of confidentiality. Fidelity is not the basic principle of morality or the controlling metaphor for the healing relationship, but it comes into play when people make agreements; the duties associated with fidelity are a function of the nature of relationships and the expectations brought to them.

**Food, Drug and Cosmetic Act of 1938.** Federal legislation providing (among other things) controls on new drugs being introduced to the market, their ingredients, labeling, and directions for use. The responsibility for preparing adequate directions for use, warnings against use, unsafe dosages, or duration of administration "necessary for the protection of users" rested with the manufacturers of these drugs.

***General Report of the Pharmaceutical Survey* (1950).** An eleven-part survey conducted between 1946 and 1949, supplemented by five monographs and special reports, the most comprehensive and most influential survey ever conducted on pharmacy practice and education in the United States. The deeply probing report concluded that "the outstanding factor determining the future of the profession of pharmacy is fundamentally moral in nature."

**"Handmaiden of the physician."** A phrase used with pride by pharmacists during the first three decades of the twentieth century to describe their subordinate professional service relationship to physicians.

**Hedonism.** The pursuit of or devotion to pleasure, especially of the senses; the belief that pleasure of happiness is the highest good. An ethical doctrine holding that only what is pleasant or has pleasant consequences is intrinsically good.

**HHS.** The Department of Health and Human Services, a successor to the Department of Health, Education and Welfare (HEW). HHS disburses most federal monies for health care and oversees federally funded medical research.

**Hippocratic Oath.** A traditional oath of ethical conduct taken by physicians upon entering into the practice of medicine. The core ethic for the Oath is the physician's pledge to act "for the benefit of the sick" within a physician-patient relationship, committing physicians to cure disease, relieve pain, or restore function, "according to my ability and judgment." For this reason, the Oath has been judged paternalistic.

**HMO.** Health maintenance organization. An insurance plan that actually delivers, and therefore, controls the health care it provides its patrons. HMOs come in many versions and are a type of managed care.

**Hospice.** An interdisciplinary program of palliative care and support services for terminally ill patients and their families. The emphasis is on comforting the dying rather than on using techniques and technologies to extend the patient's life. The care may be provided at home or in a hospice center.

**IEC.** Institutional ethics committee. A committee organized in a health care institution to assist providers, patients, and families with ethical issues associated with health care. This committee is often simply called the "ethics committee."

**Induction.** In moral philosophy, induction is the reasoning process that uses the prevailing particular moral judgments in a society to generate the general principles and rules that serve as obligatory action-guides. See **Deduction.**

**Intuitionism.** An ethical theory maintaining that our basic ethical principles are cognitive, genuine propositions capable of being judged "true" or "false." Ethical judgments are intuitive or self-evident, but are not factual and cannot be justified by empirical observation, argument, or reasoning; they are known only through intuition, direct insight, or perception.

**IPA.** Independent practice associations. Associations of physicians maintaining their independent practices while contracting with managed care organizations.

**IRB.** Institutional review board. The federally mandated review committee that any institution (such as a hospital or HMO) must have for the protection of human subjects (including fetuses) in medical research if the institution is receiving federal funding.

**IVF.** In vitro fertilization. The fertilization of an ovum in a laboratory. The term is sometimes used in a general way to designate any kind of medically assisted fertilization involving ovum retrieval.

**Justice.** An action-guiding moral principle that obliges us to treat those who are equal, in relevant respects, in the same manner. When individuals are unequal, in relevant respects, the obligation is to treat them in a fair manner. This means that those who have greater need may justly receive more of a particular resource than those with less need. Under the utilitarian concept of justice, given that available health resources are limited, in order to meet the goal of equality of health care, society is morally obligated to provide a decent minimum of health care to all claimants.

**Legal rights.** Valid claims recognized by the legal system. The rules and regulations of any legal system confer legal rights upon those subject to that system. Legal rights arise from application of some legal rule to a particular case or an appeal to legal principles (in cases where no valid legal rule implies any clear decision).

**Life-sustaining treatment.** Treatment directed primarily at preserving life despite the disease rather than at curing the disease. Ventilators, feeding tubes, dialysis, and cardiopulmonary resuscitation are primarily life-sustaining treatments, while chemotherapy is a treatment directed at primarily curing disease. A patient's decision to forgo treatment correctly believed to be life-sustaining which will result in the patient's death is often classified in legal decisions as a justified exercise in self-determination rather than suicide.

**Linda M. Strand.** Professor of Pharmacy Practice at the University of Minnesota College of Pharmacy. One of the early proponents of pharmaceutical care as a philosophy of professional pharmacy practice.

**Managed care.** A generic term encompassing a variety of prepaid and managed fee-for-service health care programs characterized by the structuring of health care around the principles associated with effective administration. Managed care programs are structured to encourage greater control over the uses and costs of health services by providing appropriate incentives and barriers for providers and their enrolled population of consumers to contain costs, manage the population and its use of services, and facilitate the paperwork required on the part of the population.

**MCO.** Managed care organization. An organization operating under the auspices of a an insurance company which has the goal of offering health services at lower costs and curbing unnecessary expenses by requiring medical procedures (except emergency care) to be approved in advance by the insurance company. Identified medical procedures require a second opinion and are subject to a utilization review process which determines how long a patient can be hospitalized.

**Medicaid.** A medical care program enacted into law in 1965 as Title XIX of the Social Security Act, jointly funded by federal and state monies and administered by individual states under broad federal guidelines to provide medical assistance to the poor, specific groups of low-income individuals, and the "categorically needy." The program provides inpatient and outpatient services, physician services, prescriptions, and laboratory work in hospitals, skilled nursing facilities, and long-term care facilities.

**Medicare.** A federally funded and administered social health insurance program for the elderly enacted into law in 1965 as Title XVIII of the Social Security Act to provide inpatient hospital and skill nursing facility care, home health care, and hospice case ("Part A") and physician services, ambulatory surgical services, and outpatient services ("Part B") to persons 65 years old and older, disabled individuals entitled to Social Security Benefits, and patients with end-stage renal disease.

**Moral dilemma.** A situation where there are two equally justifiable courses of action or judgments and the individual is uncertain which one to pursue or choose.

**Moral philosophy.** The philosophy dealing with principles of morality; an older term for ethics.

**Moral rights.** Rights grounded in natural law or moral rules commanded by God which are self-evident to human reason and independent of human beliefs or practices. Moral rights are valid claims derived from customs, traditions, and ideals which may be upheld or protected by the law. Moral rights have traditionally been correlated with the duties of justice, in contrast with the duties of charity that are not owed to any particular individual. *Institutional rights* are those rights conferred by some sort of organization or social convention.

**Natural rights.** Natural or human rights provided by social institutions which are considered to be moral claims enjoyed by all human beings by virtue of being human. Three major natural rights are the rights to life, liberty, and property.

**NIH.** The National Institutes of Health, agencies which sponsor most of the government-funded medical research in the United States.

**Nonconsequentialism.** An ethical perspective that maintains that some human actions are right or wrong no matter what the consequences. Moral values such as truthfulness and justice are pure and ideal, which when followed will result in a quality human experience without regard to consequences. Another term for **Deontology.**

**Nonmaleficence.** An action-guiding moral principle that asserts an obligation not to inflict harm on others intentionally or to engage in actions with foreseeable harmful effects. It is one of the first directives of clinical practice, expressed by the Latin maxim *primum non nocere*, "first, do no harm." Nonmaleficence complements the principle of beneficence, which requires health-care professionals to promote good.

**Nostrum.** Derived from the Latin *nostrum remedium*, "our remedy." A medicine whose effectiveness is unproved and whose ingredients are usually kept secret; a quack remedy.

**Palliative care.** Palliative care is the active total care of terminally ill patients whose disease is not responsive to curative treatment through the control of pain and other symptoms and by providing support for psychological, social, and spiritual problems, allowing death to come naturally. The goal of palliative care is achievement of the best possible quality of life for patients and their families, allowing dying patients to organize the end of their lives, participate in planning for their families' future, and help their families deal directly with death.

**Partial-birth abortion.** A procedure used in some late-term abortions whereby the lower body of a viable or periviable fetus is pulled out of the uterus and its life intentionally ended. Because maternal mortality associated with late-term abortions is significantly higher than at childbirth, the United States Supreme Court reasoned in *Roe v. Wade*, 410 US 113 (1973) that the state is required to provide much greater protection to both mother and fetus during this period and thus the state has the right to regulate and restrict a woman's ability to have an induced abortion during the third trimester.

**PAS.** Physician-assisted suicide. A form of suicide in which a physician prescribes a lethal dose of medication to a terminally ill patient or one suffering intense pain and anguish from a chronic debilitating disease who administers the fatal dose. Proponents of physician-assisted suicide argue that persons should have the right to control their own destiny, including the right to control how they die; opponents point to the principle of nonmaleficence, arguing that taking a life is harmful by definition. Also referred to as physician-assisted death (PAD).

**Paternalism.** Acts or practices that restrict or override the autonomy or known preferences of individuals without their explicit consent to benefit those individuals or to prevent harm occurring to them. Paternalistic actions may be morally justified when the benefits realized are great and the harms avoided are significant.

**Patient's Bill of Rights.** A document developed by the American Hospital Association in 1973 to serve as a guide to physicians and its members to achieve greater patient satisfaction as part of the healing process. Updated in 1992, the Bill of Rights recognize that health care is an intimate and personal interaction, and that it is incumbent upon health-care organizations and providers to understand the unique trust that patients place in them. In 1999, the Clinton administration identified the Bill of Rights as a minimum standard of care for all Americans.

**Patient-centered service.** Organizing medical, pharmaceutical, nursing, and other health-care around the needs of individual patients rather than around institutional goals.

**Pharmaceutical care.** That component of pharmacy practice which entails the direct interaction of the pharmacist with the patient with the purpose of caring for that patient's drug-related needs; the responsible provision of drug therapy for the purpose of achieving definite outcomes that improve a patient's quality of life.

**Pharmacy ethics.** The philosophical analysis of the moral phenomena found in pharmacy practice, the moral language and ethical foundations of pharmacy practice, the ethical judgments made by pharmacists, and proposals made about the normative aims and content of pharmacy practice.

**Pharmacy Patient's Bill of Rights.** A document developed by the National Association of Boards of Pharmacy in 1992 to delineate the patient's rights and responsibilities with respect to appropriate drug therapy and the patient's responsibilities and the pharmacist's rights with respect to the quality of professional services provided.

*Physicians' Drug Reference.* A compilation of drug monographs as supplied by the manufacturer; commonly referred to as the "PDR."

**PPO.** Preferred provider organization. A managed care organization with a list of preferred providers that allows patients to seek care from providers not on the list if they pay some of the cost.

**Premoral evil.** The term used by some theologians to designate bad things that are not morally evil. Killing someone is a premoral evil—it destroys human life—but is not a moral evil unless done intentionally without an adequate reason.

**Principle.** In most modern moral philosophies, a principle is an action-guide derived from an ethical theory or from experience. Moral principles (such as justice and veracity) understood as action-guides imply moral behavior governed by principles and rules.

**Principilism.** An approach to biomedical ethics through four moral principles (autonomy, nonmaleficence, beneficence, and justice), derived from actual practice, which have been refined by reflection and experience and which are open to further revision and reinterpretation in light of new cases. Often called "applied ethics," this approach to biomedical ethics was developed by scholars at the Kennedy Institute of Ethics at Georgetown University.

*Pro bono.* Derived from the Latin *pro bono publico*, "for the public good." A term often used by professions to denote the altruistic provision of services or goods without compensation for the benefit of others.

**Professional ethic.** Norms of professional practice and obligations established by a profession, usually articulated through a code of ethics developed and adopted by one or more professional associations representing that profession.

**Professional values.** Moral and nonmoral beliefs, attitudes, and standards that are derived from one's professional group.

**Prudence.** The exercise of good judgment and common sense, especially in the context of practical matters, implying not only caution but also the capacity for judging in advance the probable results of one's actions; the intellectual virtue of practical reasoning managing our natural inclinations so they enhance our life and happiness. Natural inclinations managed well are moral virtues.

**PSDA.** The Patient Self-Determination Act. A federal law, part of the Omnibus Budget Reconciliation Act (OBRA) of 1990 (42 USCA §135), effective since 1991, requiring all health-care institutions receiving federal funds to provide written information to patients about their right to make health-care decisions and providing increased weight to decisions made and acknowledged by patients through advance medical directives, including the living will and durable powers of attorney for health care.

**PVS.** Persistent vegetative state. An enduring state of total unconsciousness in which a body functions entirely in terms of its internal controls maintaining temperature, heartbeat, pulmonary ventilation, digestion, muscle reflex activity, and low-level conditioned responses with no behavioral indications of either self-awareness or awareness of surroundings. Most cases of PVS are actually permanent; all consciousness has been irreversibly lost and only a vegetative body remains. Also called "persistent unconscious state" or PUS.

*Raison d'être*. From the French *raison d'être*, "reason to be." A reason or justification for being or existing.

**Rational choice strategy.** A decision-making strategy that recommends comparing the benefits and burdens of all options simultaneously or serially before making a choice.

**Rights.** A just claim or title; that which is due to someone. *Political, civil,* or *contractual* rights are claims enjoyed by human beings by virtue of their membership in a political or civil society, or through a contract. *Institutional rights* are conferred by an organization or social convention; *moral rights* are conferred by moral grounds independent of human beliefs and practices. A *positive right* implies a positive duty to do some sort of action; a *negative right* imposes a negative duty not to act in a certain manner. For example, one who has medical insurance has the positive right to be reimbursed for medical expenses while all patients have a negative right not to be operated on without their consent. The language of rights has been a powerful influence in elevating moral consciousness and securing respect for human beings.

**Robert M. Veatch.** An early and outspoken advocate of applied ethics for the health professions. See **Principilism.**

**Situational ethics.** A method of ethical problem-solving proposed in 1979 by Joseph Fletcher who postulated that moral judgments are made by following one of two choices: *rule ethics*, which involve what one ought to do, and *situational ethics*, in which an individual judges what is best to do under the circumstances and make a decision.

**Slippery-slope argument.** An argument that claims a proposal is not really morally objectionable in itself but should be rejected because it will inevitably, or almost inevitably, lead to morally objectionable actions. The argument is once you take the first step on a slippery slope, you will not be able to prevent sliding down into a moral abyss. Also known as the "wedge argument" or the "camel's nose argument."

**Social justice.** A contractual approach to justice found in the works of Immanuel Kant who claimed that a civil state ought to be founded on an original contract satisfying three requirements: *freedom* to seek happiness in whatever way one sees fit as long as one does not infringe upon the freedom of others to pursue a similar end; *equality*, the right of each person to restrict others from using their freedom in ways that deny freedom to all; and *independence*, which is presupposed for each person by the free agreement to the original contract.

**Social contracts.** A model of society based on seventeenth-century social contract theory in which a society is constituted by individuals for the fulfillment of individual ends, with social goods as aggregates of private goods. Critics claim that this vision of life and society ignores aspects of community life, such as reciprocal obligation and mutual independence, eroding the bases of authority in family and polity alike.

**Stoicism.** An ancient school of philosophy that assimilated law and morality which maintained that all nature, including human nature, is structured and functions in a rational way; hence, our moral task is to live according to nature, balancing organic needs (such as eating, drinking, and pleasure) with rational control (transforming our organic needs and impulses). Stoic physicians might refuse to provide pain relief to suffering patients because they believed that patients should be allowed to suffer for their own good in order to strengthen their characters and powers of resolution.

**Surrogate.** The person making a decision on behalf of a person without decision-making capacity. Surrogate is another term for proxy.

**Teleology.** Any moral philosophy based on outcome or end result. The most popular modern teleological theory is *utilitarianism*. See **Utilitarianism** and, for contrast, **Deontology**.

**Terminal sedation.** The use of a sedative to make a patient unconscious when treatment is withdrawn.

**Therapeutic misadventure.** A term coined by Henri R. Manasse, Jr., in 1989 to describe medication-related morbidity or morality associated with the way drugs are prescribed, dispensed, and used, problems which are not inherent in the drugs themselves.

**TPN.** Total parenteral nutrition; nutrition meeting all body requirements inserted into the venous system rather that the gastrointestinal tract.

**Triage.** Originally the prioritizing of scarce resources in an emergency by organizing the injured into three groups: those who can do without the resources for now, those who will probably not benefit from the resources, and those who will benefit from the resources and need them to survive. Triage has come to mean screening patients on their immediate medical needs and directing them to appropriate care, such as an emergency room, an urgent care center, or a physician's office. Triage usually takes places in circumstances of temporary crisis which require quick decisions about the critical care of a pool of patients. Generally, these decisions are controlled by utilitarian considerations.

**Truthfulness.** Veracity, being truthful, habitually telling the truth. The virtues of candor and truthfulness are among the most widely praised character traits of health professionals in contemporary biomedical ethics. Truthfulness draws its strength from the complex support it provides to diverse values—respecting others, avoiding coercion and manipulation, supporting community, maintain reciprocity in relationships, supporting the value of communication, eliminating the costs and complexities of deception, refraining from unduly assuming responsibility, and maintaining trust. See **Veracity.**

**UDDA.** Uniform Determination of Death Act. A statute written by the National Conference of Commissioners on Uniform State Laws, this act serves as a model for defining two criteria of death—the cardiopulmonary criterion and the brain-dead criterion. An individual who is "brain dead" has sustained either irreversible cessation of circulatory and respiratory functions or irreversible cessation of all functions of the entire brain, including the brain stem.

**Unethical behavior.** Individual or collective behavior that knowingly and willingly violates fundamental norms of ethical conduct toward others.

**Unprofessional conduct.** The Medical Act of 1858, at the instigation of the newly established British Medical Association, established the General Medical Council to protect the public by controlling admission to the medical register on the basis of explicit educational and ethical standards to exclude unqualified practitioners from practicing medicine and to ensure that only those orthodox practitioners who had attained the prescribed standards were admitted to the register. Moreover, qualified medical practitioners who fell below the prescribed standards were liable to disciplinary action, including removal from the register if they were found guilty of "infamous conduction in a professional respect," performing abortions or active euthanasia, having sexual relations with patients, abusing alcohol or drugs, fee splitting, "covering" for medical practice carried out by unregistered persons, convictions in court that would bring dishonor to the profession, abuse of financial opportunities afforded by medical practice, improper denigration of professional colleagues, advertising for the physician's own financial advantage, and canvassing for patients. American standards for unprofessional conduct of both physicians and pharmacists developed from the British model.

**Utilitarianism.** The moral philosophy based on bringing about the greatest good for the largest number of individuals. The utility of an act is determined by its tendency to promote or produce happiness; the right action among alternative choices is most correct if that action produces the greatest good. In *act utilitarianism*, one analyzes the act and seeks to determine when an alternative in a particular case would maximize the opportunity for good or minimize suffering; in *rule utilitarianism*, one focuses on the effect of action and analyzes policies, asking which policy, as a general rule, would maximize happiness and minimize suffering. An alternative to **Deontology.**

**Utility.** The ultimate moral principle or law proposed by utilitarians as the origin of all morality and as the source of moral obligation. Sometimes called the "greatest happiness principle," where happiness is understood as the happiness of everyone. John Stuart Mill suggested that utility "holds that actions are right in proportion as they tend to promote happiness, wrong as they tend to promote the opposite of happiness." Utility is frequently portrayed as a specification of the normative principle of beneficence and considered a "balancing" principle in assessing harms and benefits, and is deeply embedded in debates over social priorities for health care and rationing scarce resources.

**Value.** A standard or quality that is esteemed, desired, considered important or has worth or merit. Values are expressed by behaviors or standards that a person endorses or tries to maintain. *Organic values*, such as life, health, vigor, and bodily integrity are basic to our human existence. *Moral values*, such as dignity, integrity, mutual respect, stability, effectiveness, and inclusiveness, cluster around personal identity, interpersonal relationships, the makeup of groups, associations, social institutions, societies, and even the global community. We normally discuss moral values in terms of *rights* and *duties*. Rights identify claims that others properly make on us; duties consist of *obligations* and *prohibitions*. Obligations specify what we must do no matter what else we might hope to accomplish; prohibitions specify what we must not do regardless of larger objectives. It is for the sake of moral values that basic rights and duties are binding.

**Veracity.** The moral principle that obliges one to tell the truth and to not lie or deceive others. Philosophers have generally treated veracity as an obligation flowing from more fundamental theoretical principles, such as utility, religious duty, respect for persons, or some combination of beneficence, fidelity, and autonomy. See **Truthfulness.**

**Virtue.** A disposition (such as honesty or kindness) or trait (such as conscientiousness) that is valued and is acquired in part, by teaching and practice, and, perhaps, by grace. A disposition or trait to undertake certain types of actions in certain types of situations in accordance with moral obligations or moral ideals is often called *moral virtue*. When a thing or person functions well, the Greeks called its functioning *excellent* or *virtuous*. When individuals manage their natural inclinations well they are *morally* excellent. Achieving moral excellence requires prudence, the *intellectual* excellence relevant to ethics.

# Index[*]

---

[*]References to illustrations are set in *italics*.